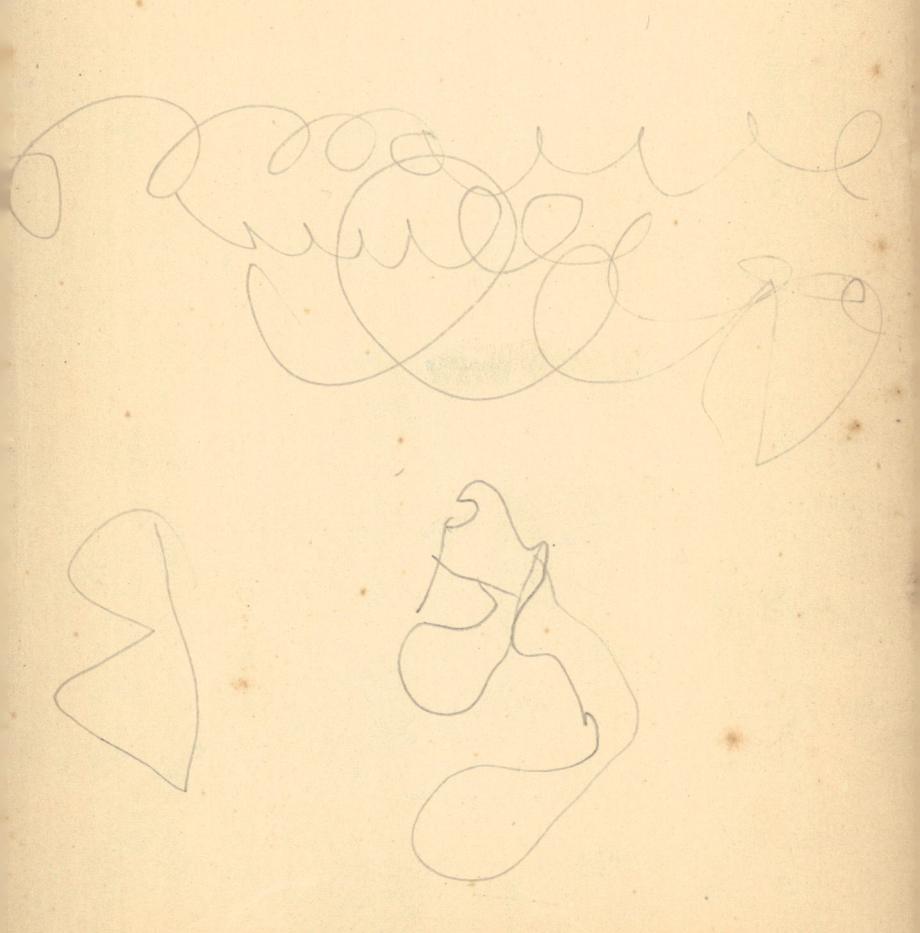

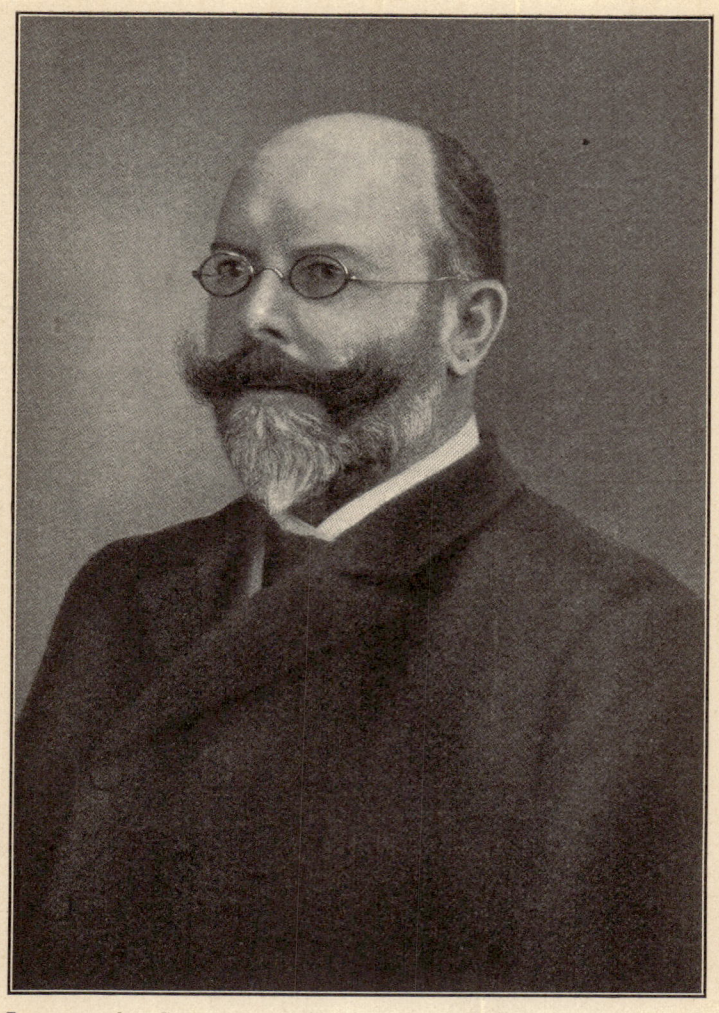

LOEFLER, the German who discovered the diphtheria germ which kills over fifty children daily in our country

THE HUMAN BODY
AND
HEALTH

AN INTERMEDIATE TEXT-BOOK OF
ESSENTIAL PHYSIOLOGY, APPLIED HYGIENE, AND
PRACTICAL SANITATION FOR SCHOOLS

BY

ALVIN DAVISON, M.S., A.M., Ph.D.

PROFESSOR OF BIOLOGY IN LAFAYETTE COLLEGE

INTERMEDIATE

NEW YORK :: CINCINNATI :: CHICAGO
AMERICAN BOOK COMPANY

Copyright, 1909, by
ALVIN DAVISON
Entered at Stationers' Hall, London

HUMAN BODY. INT.

W. P. I

PREFACE

A few minutes' reflection in regard to the modern ways of living will fix in the mind of any sound reasoner the conviction that we are a careless and cruel people. Nearly 1000 human beings in the United States are dying daily of diseases which science has shown how to prevent. Streams are polluted, garbage dumped on the nearest vacant lot, fresh air and sunshine shut out of the houses by double doors and windows, and innocent children fed dirty milk because people do not realize that these acts are responsible for many of the 4000 graves daily made in our nation's cemeteries.

Sanitary science and the public health can be advanced only as they are supported by an intelligent public opinion. Laws necessary to the public welfare can be secured and upheld when the majority of citizens appreciate the value of the problems involved. New ideas are grasped most readily by the young and it is with them that modern hygienic teaching will have the greatest influence. Parents do not recognize that eyesight is being impaired, normal growth prevented, blood poisoned, and the body starved because of customs and habits born in ignorance.

An effort has been made to present in this book the subject of personal and public health in such a way as to appeal to the interest of boys and girls and fix in their minds the essentials of right living. Knowing anatomy and physiology is of little value to our young folks unless it helps them to practice intelligently in their daily lives the teachings of hygiene and sanitation.

In place of general statements in regard to promoting health, specific facts and full explanations are given showing how disease is caused and how the body may be kept well and strong. Much labor and expense have been devoted to the preparation of the illustrations which the pupils should be required to study carefully.

A few experiments have been outlined and many other experiments and helpful suggestions for the teacher are given in the Advanced book of this series. The importance of proving the truth and making clear the leading facts relating to efficient living, by simple demonstrations and experiments cannot be overestimated.

Every teacher is urged to secure from the State Board of Health, at the capital of the state, copies of the numerous bulletins issued concerning health. These are sent free to those requesting them. The teacher who does her duty in imparting instruction that invites health and happiness will bless not only those of to-day, but generations yet unborn.

CONTENTS

CHAPTER		PAGE
I.	The Human Body as a Living Machine	9
II.	Plants and Animals Related to Health	13
III.	The Plan of the Human Body	21
IV.	Food for the Body	27
V.	The Care and Cooking of Food	36
VI.	How Food is used by the Body	42
VII.	Drink and Health	60
VIII.	Tobacco and Other Narcotics and their Effect on Health	71
IX.	The Blood and its Passage through the Body	78
X.	Breathing and its Use	95
XI.	Air and Health	103
XII.	Cleanliness and Warmth	113
XIII.	Clothing and Colds	127
XIV.	The Bones	133
XV.	The Muscles and Exercise	143
XVI.	How the Body is Governed	153
XVII.	The Care of the Nervous System and how Narcotics Affect it	165

CHAPTER		PAGE
XVIII.	Organs for Receiving Knowledge	174
XIX.	The Cause of Sickness	188
XX.	How to Keep Well	200
	Pronunciation and Explanation of Difficult Words	215
	Index	219

THE HUMAN BODY AND HEALTH

CHAPTER I

THE HUMAN BODY AS A LIVING MACHINE

The Body like a Locomotive.—The locomotive moves about and does work at the bidding of the engineer. It does this just as long as it is supplied with water, and coal or wood, if the ashes, the burnt waste matters, are removed, and if its parts are kept in order.

No engineer is trusted to manage a locomotive until he understands all its parts and how they work. To avoid wrecks and loss of life, he must examine his machine at the end of every trip and see that every screw, lever and wheel is in proper order.

The human body is in many ways like the locomotive and each person is his own engineer. The body does what its owner commands as long as it is fed, if the ashes, the waste matters, are removed and if its parts are kept in a healthy condition.

Why One should know the Parts of the Body.—No railroad company will trust the management of a locomotive to an engineer who does not know its parts, because by the neglect to repair a weak or worn part the entire engine may be ruined. For the same reason every person, who is the engineer of his own body, should know its parts.

The study of the parts of the body and their location is called *anatomy*. The greatest use of anatomy is to help one to understand how the parts of the body do their work.

Learning the Use of the Parts.—The engineer must understand the use of each lever, wheel and screw in his engine in order to determine when they are in proper working condition. A person must likewise know the use of the various parts of his body to understand when they are doing their work properly.

The use of any certain portion of the body is spoken of as its *function*. The study of the function of the heart, lungs or other parts of the body is known as *physiology*.

One of the chief benefits to be had from the study of physiology is the knowledge which aids us much in understanding how to care for the body. By proper care all its parts may be kept in a healthy state and in most cases sickness may be prevented.

Taking Care of the Body.—The body is a much more delicate machine than the locomotive. It is often injured by food taken at the wrong time, or in too large quantities. Impure oil and dirty coal sometimes clog parts of the locomotive and make it do poor work. Impure air and unclean food and water often seriously damage the human body so as to cause sickness and even death.

The study of the care of the body and of how to prevent fevers, colds and ill health of all sorts is called *hygiene*. Happiness and health depend largely upon hygiene.

Importance of Hygiene.—During the eighteenth century, it is estimated that 50,000,000 persons died of smallpox in Europe. To-day the disease is so uncommon that many physicians have never seen a case.

Scurvy which afflicted so many of the sailors a century or two ago now seldom occurs because the men have learned what kind of food to eat to avoid the disease. Of the French soldiers who went to fight the people of Madagascar, seven thousand died of fevers which we now know how to prevent, and only twenty-nine were killed in battle. In our war with Spain, less than three hundred of our soldiers were killed in battle, but over three thousand died of disease which hygiene has shown how to avoid.

What Hygiene does.—Hygiene protects the body in time of peace as the shield and steel armor of the old Romans protected them in time of war. Health depends largely upon preventing tiny plants and animals called germs, from feeding upon our bodies, and upon supplying the body with the proper food, air, drink and clothing.

Among every thousand people there are more than twice as many deaths yearly in Russia and India as in Sweden. This is because the Russians and people of India do not observe the teachings of hygiene so carefully as the Swedes. In London, a hundred years ago, the number of deaths in every thousand residents was three times as great as in the year 1900.

Why All should know Hygiene.—In order that we may be a healthy nation, every one must observe the laws of hygiene. Each person by his own efforts alone may not be able to protect his health, for the ignorant may furnish him bad food or bad water. A milkman caused 236 cases of diphtheria in one city by being so careless as to help care for the milk when he was recovering from diphtheria. One hundred years ago, the average length of human life in the United States was 28 years. Hygiene has shown us how to prevent sickness and death so that the average length of life is now 42 years.

1500-1600	1600-1700	1700-1800	1800-1850	1850-1900	1900-1910
15 acres	14 acres	13 acres	11 acres	8 acres	7 acres

FIG. 1—Number of acres required yearly to bury the dead among each 1,000,000 inhabitants in Germany, England and the United States. Note that the number of deaths is decreasing as people learn how to avoid disease.

Practical Questions

1. In what way is the body like a locomotive? 2. Why should a person know much about his body? 3. What is meant by anatomy? 4. Of what use is anatomy? 5. Why should you know the use of the parts of the body? 6. What is physiology? 7. How does the study of physiology benefit one? 8. Describe what is meant by hygiene? 9. Name some diseases which long ago killed many. 10. Upon what does health depend? 11. Why do more people die in some countries than in others? 12. Why can one not protect his health by his efforts alone? 13. How can we secure the best health as a nation?

CHAPTER II

PLANTS AND ANIMALS RELATED TO HEALTH

Bacteria.—Bacteria are also called *microbes* or *germs*. There are hundreds of kinds of bacteria and all are so small that a million together would not make a mass so large as the head of a pin. They are of various shapes. Most of them are straight, curved, or twisted rods. Some have the form of a ball.

Bacteria occur nearly everywhere. A bit of dirt as large as a pea may contain a million bacteria, and a hundred thousand of them are commonly present in a cup of water. More than a million bacteria are lodged on the surface of the body and billions dwell in the mouth and intestine.

Many kinds of bacteria are useful, but a few kinds sometimes cause serious disease when they grow in other plants, or in the bodies of animals or man.

Nature of Bacteria.—A hundred years ago many people thought that dead matter could of itself change into living plants or animals. When meat broth is put away in the cupboard for a day or two, the microscope shows it to be full of tiny forms of life. It is now known that this life does not start from the broth, but consists of bacteria. They are constantly floating through the air and can be kept out of food by placing it in airtight jars. The food and the jars must first be boiled to kill the bacteria in them. The spoiling or souring of food of any kind is generally due to bacteria.

Need of Bacteria.—Experiment shows that higher life depends upon the help of bacteria. The dead leaves, grass, fallen trees and the waste matter of the barnyard cannot rot or decay without the aid of bacteria. If these little plants were destroyed, the surface of the earth would soon become covered with dead matter.

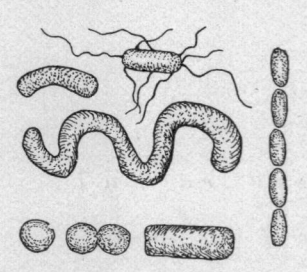

FIG. 2.—Harmless bacteria so numerous in drinking water that a person often takes a half-million into his stomach daily. Much enlarged.

These ever-present bacteria change the dead plants and animals and all other waste products of life into a food which the new plants can use the next season. Some bacteria feed upon living animals instead of dead matter. It is these that cause disease.

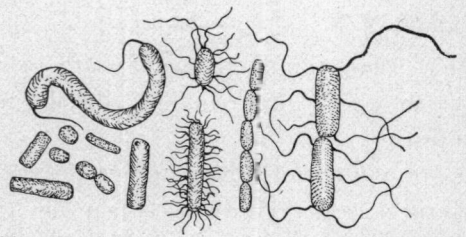

FIG. 3.—Useful bacteria which change dead matter into food for the grass, wheat and corn. Much enlarged.

Bacteria of Disease.—Fifty million persons are every

year forced to the sick bed in this country and Europe by bacteria. Each disease is caused by a certain kind of germs and if these are kept out of the body, the sickness cannot occur.

Some of the common diseases resulting from bacteria are *pneumonia, measles, typhoid fever, diphtheria, sore throat,*

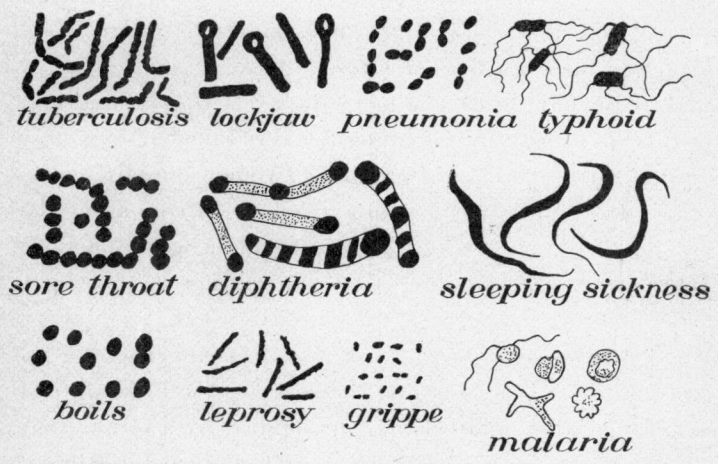

FIG. 4.—The germs causing various diseases. Much enlarged.

grippe and *tuberculosis*. When the germs of these diseases get into the body, they devour the tissues and give off poisons.

How Bacteria get into the Body.—Bacteria nearly always enter the body through the mouth. The germs of typhoid fever generally reach the system with water which has received the waste matter from a typhoid patient. The bacteria of pneumonia, sore throat, diphtheria and grippe are frequently received from the drinking cup, pencils or other objects used by persons recently recovered from these diseases. The germs are sometimes breathed in with dust. The bacteria of tuberculosis reach the body with air or food or are scraped from the drinking cup or other objects used by the sick.

If nurses and patients would be careful to destroy with boiling water or formalin the germs which leave the bodies of the sick in the spit and other excretions, there would be fewer bacteria to make people sick.

How Bacteria grow.—When supplied with food and kept warm, bacteria grow very rapidly. Cold makes them grow more slowly. One plant produces two new ones by separating in the middle. This can occur every fifteen minutes so that one germ can produce millions in a single day.

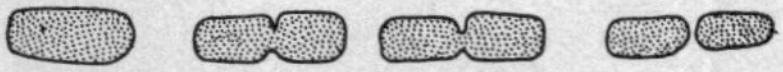

FIG. 5.—Drawing of a germ at intervals of ten minutes while growing.

In some bacteria deprived of food and moisture, the contents of the plant collect in one part and become surrounded by a tough coat. This part with its coat is a *spore*. Boiling water will kill most spores in less than ten minutes. Our common disease bacteria do not have spores and therefore they are killed by being boiled one minute.

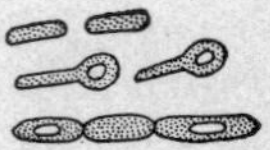

FIG. 6.—Bacteria. The white bodies are spores.

Mold.—Mold belongs to the group of plants known as fungi. They have no light green coloring matter in them and cannot feed on the air as plants with green leaves do.

Mold often forms white or greenish patches on bread or fruit in a damp cellar. It is made of fine threads from which other hairlike branches stick up into the air. These branches bear on their ends little knobs containing dozens of tiny balls called *spores*. These spores break loose and float about in the dust. When they fall upon moist food they sprout and grow into a patch of mold. The spores are hard to kill but eight minutes in boiling water will usually cause their death.

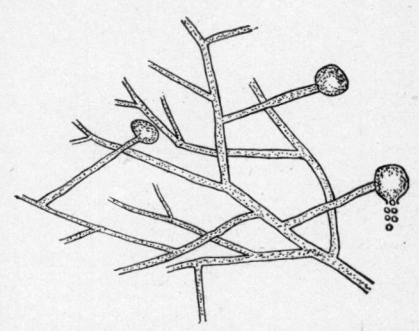

FIG. 7.—Bread mold much enlarged. Note the tiny spores bursting from their case in the right upper corner.

Some kinds of mold grow on the body and cause disease. *Barber's itch* and *ringworm* are caused by molds growing in the skin. The spores are carried from one face to another by the uncleaned razor, towel or brush. Other diseases are sometimes caught by using soiled towels in public places.

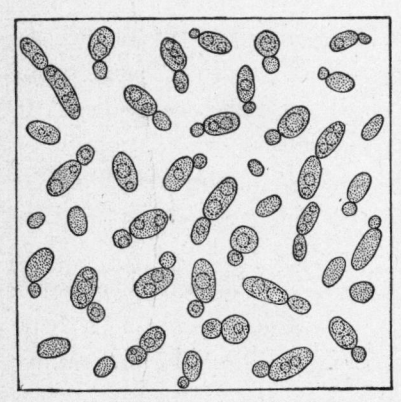

FIG. 8.—Yeast plants much enlarged. Note the bud at the end in several plants about to form a new plant.

Yeast.—This is a tiny round plant too small to be seen without the microscope. It is common on fruit. One kind of yeast is used in making bread. It changes the sugar in the dough into alcohol and a gas. The gas pushes apart the particles of dough and makes it light.

Yeast is also used in making beer, wine, whisky and other alcoholic drinks which often cause much ill health and unhappiness. It is the yeast plant which gets into cider and makes it work or turn sour. The biting taste is due to the alcohol and carbon dioxide.

Animal Parasites.—Any plant or animal which feeds upon another living plant or animal without at once destroying it, is a *parasite*. The bacteria of disease are all parasites. Some animals live in the human body and produce disease. Yellow fever, sleeping sickness and malaria are caused by tiny animals which get into the body by the bite of a fly or mosquito. The plague which has killed millions of people in Asia and some in our own country is caused by bacteria, but the germs are usually put beneath the skin by the bite of bugs or fleas which have been sucking blood from sick persons or from rats.

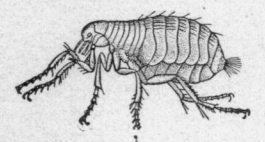

FIG. 9.—A flea which carries the germs of plague from the sick to the well.

The Itch Mite and Head Lice.—The *itch* was once a very common disease. When it was discovered that a little spider living in the skin was the cause of the continuous itching, a way of killing it was soon found (Fig. 10). The disease is now easily cured by an ointment which any physician can supply.

Tiny six-legged insects called *head lice* sometimes live among the hair. They cause continuous itching and sleeplessness. They are easily killed by thoroughly rubbing the scalp with equal parts of olive oil and coal oil before going to bed. The hair should then be kept from soiling the linen by wrapping a towel about the head. In the morning the head should be washed with soap and equal parts of vinegar and hot water to remove the tiny white eggs clinging to the hair. This treatment should be given two or three times.

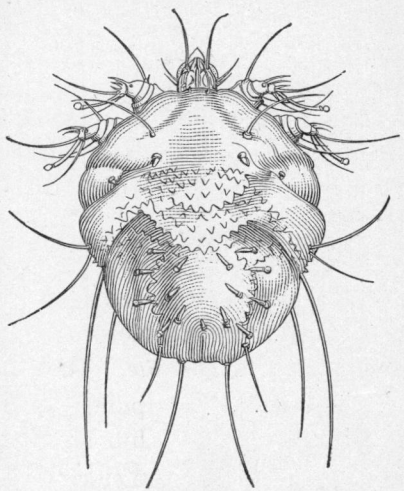

Fig. 10.—The tiny spider which causes the itch when living in the skin. Much enlarged.

Overcoming the Parasites.—Owing to the fact that many sick persons through carelessness let disease germs escape from their bodies, everybody is likely to get some of these enemies into his body. The studies of physiology and hygiene have shown that persons may prevent many of them from entering the body or even from growing after they are in the body. Prevention of the sickness which they cause, as well as of other kinds of sickness, depends much upon understanding the plan of the body, the care and use of food, and the care and use of the organs as explained in the following chapters.

Practical Questions

1. Give two other names for bacteria. 2. What is the form of bacteria? 3. Where are bacteria found? 4. When may bacteria be harmful? 5. How may bacteria be kept away from food? 6. Of what use are some bacteria? 7. State a fact showing that bacteria cause much sickness. 8. Name some diseases due to bacteria. 9. How do the germs of typhoid fever often get into the body? 10. State how the bacteria of other diseases may enter the body. 11. What should nurses and patients do to prevent sickness in other persons? 12. Describe how bacteria grow. 13. What is a spore? 14. Why are some bacteria harder to kill than others? 15. Describe mold. 16. What kinds of mold cause disease? 17. What is yeast? 18. Describe the use of yeast. 19. What is a parasite? 20. Name some diseases caused by tiny animals living in the body. 21. Why should one having itch not sit near or handle things to be used by other persons? 22. Why should one with head lice not use another person's brush or hat? 23. How can we prevent sickness from parasites?

Suggestions for the Teacher

The presence of mold germs in dust may easily be shown in the following manner: Rub a piece of bread across one board of a dusty floor and then lay it soiled-side up in a saucer containing two tablespoonfuls of water. Cover with a bowl and let it remain in a warm place from three to six days. The white threads of mold may then be seen and on the ends of the upright branches are tiny balls each containing a hundred or more spores.

CHAPTER III

THE PLAN OF THE HUMAN BODY

Nature of Living Things.—Living plants and animals differ from all dead objects such as iron and stone by being able to take food and change it so as to form a part of their own bodies. The corn plant takes in some of its food through the leaves and some through the roots. In some of the worms and other lower animals, the food in a watery state passes directly through the skin into the body. Most animals, however, have a special opening called the mouth for the purpose of receiving food, and a sac or canal in which the food is changed to a liquid. Then there are tubes for taking the food to all parts of the body and for carrying off the waste matter.

Special structures are provided for moving the body, and there are still other structures called nerves to make all parts of the body work in proper order. These several duties such as

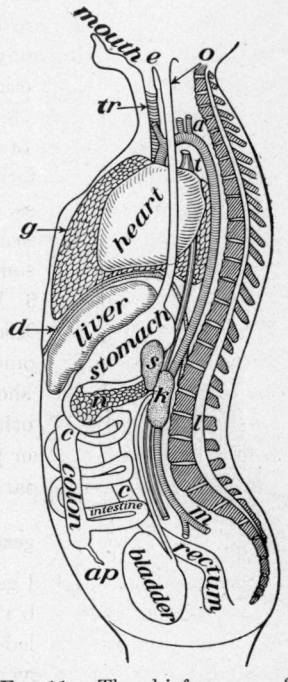

FIG. 11.—The chief organs of the body from the side. *a*, arch of the aorta or main artery of the trunk; *c*, large intestine; *d*, diaphragm; *e*, throat; *g*, lung; *k*, kidney; *l*, spinal cord within the back bone; *m*, main artery dividing to go to the legs; *n*, pancreas; *o*, gullet; *s*, spleen; *tr*, wind pipe; *t*, main vein of body; *ap*, appendix.

preparing food, carrying it about in the body and moving the body, are performed by separate portions of the human body, which are named *systems*.

The Systems.—There are eight chief systems forming the human body. The *framework* or *bony system* is for support and movement. The lean meat makes up much of the *muscular system* used in moving the bones. The mouth, stomach, intestine and whatever else helps to prepare the food for use form the *digestive system*. The blood tubes, conveying the food from the intestine to all parts of the body and carrying off the waste matter, constitute the *blood system*.

The *breathing system* consists of the lungs and other parts used in supplying the body with air. The skin and kidneys taking the waste matter out of the blood belong to the *sewer system*. The brain and nerves form the *nervous system* which directs the actions of all parts of the body.

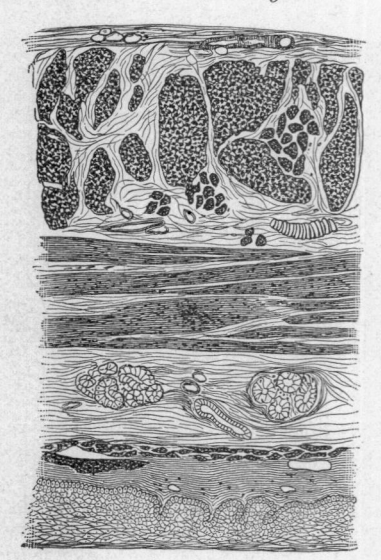

FIG. 12.—Slice of the wall of the gullet enlarged to show nature of tissues.

The Parts of a System.—Each system is composed of several parts called *organs*. Each organ has a certain work to do in helping the body to keep well and perform the duties of life. The heart is the organ for sending the blood through the body, the stomach is an organ for digesting food, and a lung is an organ for breathing.

Nature of an Organ.—The organs when examined with a microscope enlarging their parts are seen to be made of several different substances. Each of these is called a *tissue*. The stomach is lined with one kind of *tissue* while its outer part is made of *muscular tissue* (Fig. 12.) Among these two is a *nervous tissue*, and the three are bound together by a *connective tissue* made mostly of fine threads.

Parts of a Tissue.—The microscope shows that the tissues are made of *cells* mingled with fine threads or other substance. A *cell* is a tiny mass of matter containing a smaller particle of matter called the *nucleus*. Usually each cell is surrounded by a thin membrane, the *cell wall* (Fig. 13).

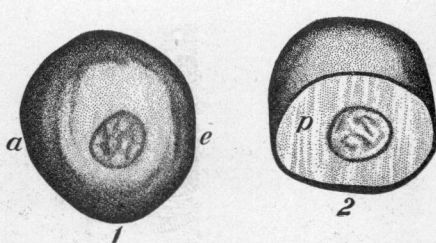

FIG. 13.—A cell much enlarged. 2 is the upper half of 1, cut through the line *a-e*. The dark spot is the nucleus.

The form of cells varies widely. The fat cells are like little balls while the muscle cells are rodlike. The nerve cells are very irregular with branching processes. Some of the cells such as those on the surface of the skin are flat like the scales of a fish and others in the intestine are shaped like tiny corks.

Character of Cells.—All plants and animals are composed of one or more cells united by threadlike fibers, or by other matter. Each of many plants and animals living in dirty

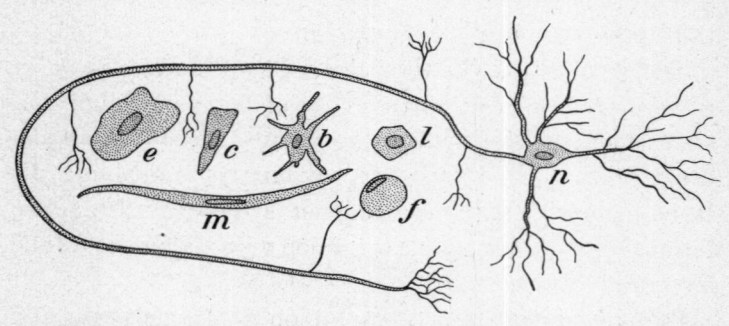

Fig. 14.—Various kinds of cells many times enlarged. *n*, from the brain; *f*, fat cell; *m*, muscle; *e*, surface of skin.

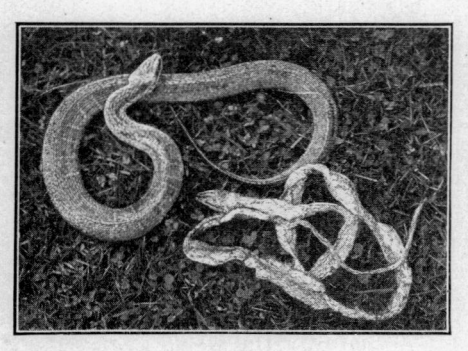

Fig. 15.—A water snake which has just shed its outer skin.

water is made of a single cell. They require food and air just the same as the cells of the body and also give off waste matter. After growing to a certain size, these animals divide in the middle and each half swims away as a new animal to repeat the process the next day. In the same way new cells are formed in the body, but instead of moving apart they stick fast together.

Dying Parts of the Body.—Dead cells can be scraped from the skin at any time. Some animals such as frogs and snakes shed the entire dead outer skin in one piece several times each year. The cells beneath divide and thus form other cells for a new skin.

The cells within the deep parts of the body remain in place year after year, but tiny bits of them are dying constantly and passing out in the breath, the sweat and in other ways. These dead bits are burned to ashes in the body in much the same way that a match burns. The burning of anything means the union with it of a part of the air called *oxygen*.

Burning or Oxidation.—The union of oxygen with any other substance is *oxidation*. The head of a match is scratched to make it hot enough to cause the oxygen of the air to unite with it.

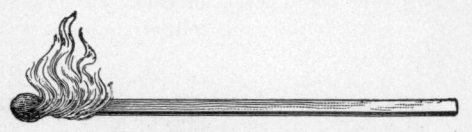

FIG. 16.—Oxidation of a match

The living action of the cells in the body makes the oxygen there unite with the dead particles and burn them into ashes so that they can be carried out of the body through the lungs and kidneys, and not clog the organs. This burning or oxidation of the dead parts of the cells, and of the food brought there by the blood, goes on very slowly so there is no flame but enough heat to keep the body warm. By experiment, it has been found that the oxidation of an ounce of fat within the body furnishes just the same amount of heat as the burning of an ounce of fat produces when burned outside of the body.

Practical Questions

1. How does dead matter differ from living things? 2. What animals do not have mouths? 3. What is a system in the body? 4. Name some of the systems in the body. 5. Tell what three of the systems are used for. 6. What is an organ? 7. Name five organs in the body. 8. What is a tissue? 9. Tell how the cells differ. 10. How do cells grow? 11. How are the dying parts of the body cast off? 12. What is oxidation? 13. What makes oxidation occur in the body? 14. What results from oxidation in the body? 15. Where is oxygen burned in the body?

Suggestions for the Teacher

The fact that parts of the body are dying and are being cast off may be shown in the following manner: Secure two or three frogs, or salamanders found in ponds or under stones near streams and place them in a jar containing a half inch of water. Generally within a week, large strips of shed skin may be seen floating in the water. The shed skins of caterpillars or other insects may often be found sticking to stones or trees. Any caterpillar confined in a box and fed for a few days with the leaves of the plant on which it was found will shed its skin.

CHAPTER IV

FOOD FOR THE BODY

Need of Food.—The body consists of about twelve gallons of water; twelve pounds of mineral matter such as table salt, potash, lime and iron; twelve pounds of fat; and twenty-four pounds of proteid. *Proteid* forms a portion of every cell in the body. A common form of proteid is *albumin* like the white of egg. Since parts of the body made of these substances are dying daily and passing away, such food must be taken as will restore the loss.

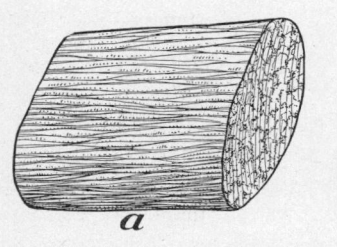

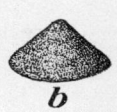

FIG. 17.—*b*, the mineral matter such as lime, salt and potash left from burning the piece of meat, *a*.

Food is also required for fuel to be burned to keep the body warm, and to supply energy to make it move and enable the organs to do their work. A steam locomotive cannot pull cars without burning coal. For the same reason, the arm or leg cannot be moved without something being burned in the body.

Kinds of Food.—The two general groups of foods are the *flesh foods* and the *fuel foods*. The flesh foods are the proteids. These form a large part of **lean meat, of** dried peas and beans, and of **wheat flour.** They help build up bone, blood, and flesh.

The *fuel foods* consist of sugars, starches, and fats. These are used to give energy for work and to keep the body warm. The sugar used on the table is made largely from beets and from sugar cane. Milk sugar is present in milk, and fruit sugar makes the ripe fruit sweet. Starch is found mainly in such vegetables as corn, rice, wheat, and potatoes, where it appears in the form of little grains (Fig. 18).

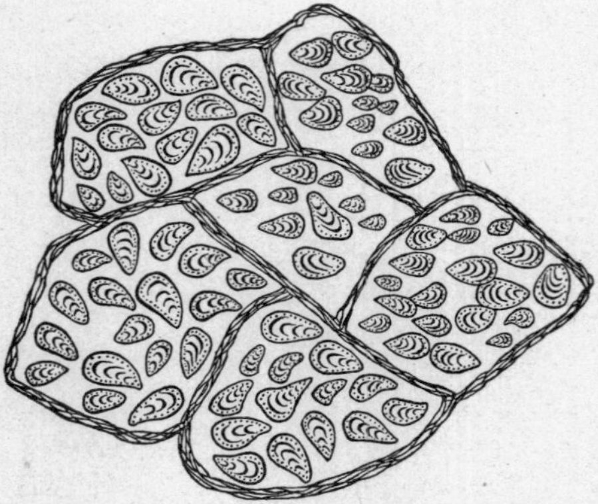

FIG. 18.—A tiny slice of potato to show the starch grains. Much enlarged.

Fats make up most of the fat meat, form a large part of the cream of milk and about nine tenths of butter. The fat of beef is called *tallow* and that from pork is known as *lard*. A fat which is liquid at room temperature is spoken of as *oil*. Cottonseed oil, castor oil and olive oil are derived from plants.

Quantity of Food Required.—Careful experiments lately made have shown that most people eat too much. No matter how much food is eaten, only that part of it required by the body for replacing worn-out material and

FOOD FOR THE BODY

furnishing fuel will be used. The extra amount eaten is likely to cause sickness by clogging the organs or by helping bacteria to develop in the food canal and to give off poisons. These produce headache and other kinds of illness called *indigestion* or *dyspepsia*.

Cost of Food.—Many foods contain much water and have a pleasant taste but there is very little solid matter present to form flesh or to supply fuel to the body. Water

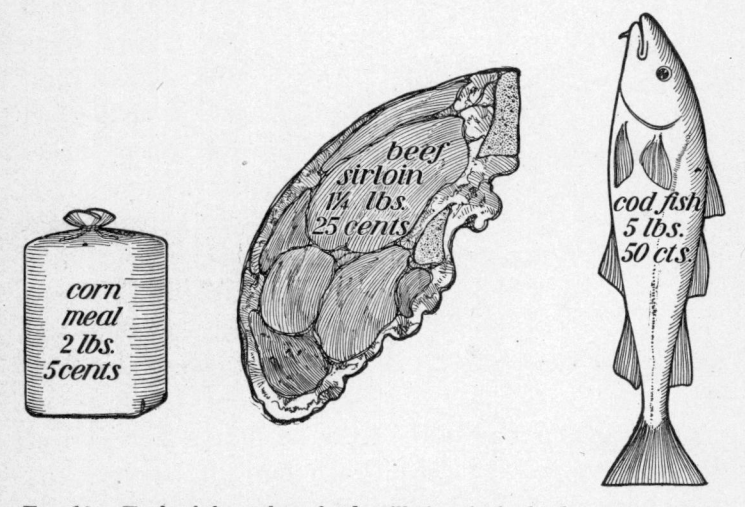

FIG. 19.—Each of these three foods will give the body the same nourishment, but the fish costs ten times as much as the corn meal.

melons, cucumbers, oysters, lobsters, bananas, cabbages and apples are *expensive foods* as they contain little nourishment.

Wheat flour, corn meal, and potatoes are *cheap foods*. They are rich in flesh and fuel making power. Ten cents' worth of corn meal will furnish as much nourishment as two dollars worth of oysters. A dime spent for stewing beef will secure more food value than twenty-five cents spent for sirloin steak.

How to Live Cheaply.—Good food can be secured for a small amount of money if the housekeeper is careful to purchase what contains the most nourishment for the least cost. The daily cost of food for a family of five persons living largely upon wheat bread, corn meal mush, beef stew, small dried beans, potatoes, oatmeal and two quarts of milk, with a little of the cheapest fruit and green vegetables in season, need not exceed seventy-five cents.

Meats.—The eating of large quantities of meat is responsible for much ill health. Intemperance in the use of meat and alcohol is one of the important causes of disease of the kidneys. Those who live much indoors should not use pork or fried meats more than once or twice weekly. Baked fish and roasted or boiled beef or mutton should be eaten only once daily by those taking little exercise.

The same nourishment supplied by meats may be purchased for less money spent for eggs, milk and vegetables. Sirloin, round, and rump steaks are expensive cuts and furnish but little more nourishment than chuck or brisket costing one third as much (Fig. 23).

Eggs.—Eggs contain much substance for the making of flesh and also a considerable amount of fat. They form an excellent food especially for invalids, and children over nine months old They are most easily digested when beaten raw in a glass of milk. Soft-boiled eggs are also easily digested.

FOOD FOR THE BODY 31

One dozen eggs furnish about the same amount of nourishment as a pound of beef sirloin.

Milk.—The one food of more importance than any other for man's welfare is milk. Seven eighths of it consists of water but the other eighth contains all the elements needed for the body. Anyone can live for years upon milk alone, but for adults it is more useful when taken with other foods.

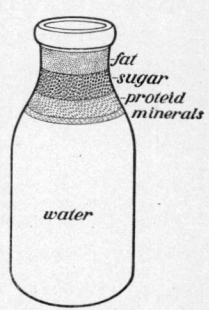

Milk is easily digested and is, therefore, an excellent food for children and invalids. It contains much mineral matter for making bones and is rich in other substances needed to form flesh and blood. Three or four glasses of milk may be used daily by most children with marked benefit. It should not be swallowed rapidly like water, but taken slowly in sips. When taken cold it may not agree with some persons. It should then be sipped slowly while very hot. In heating it, do not let it boil.

FIG. 20.—A bottle of milk showing of what it is made. Proteid is the flesh building food.

Boiled milk should not be used regularly unless a physician directs it. One or two quarts of clean milk taken daily is a great help both in preventing and curing tuberculosis. Milk at six cents per quart would be a cheap food. Two quarts of milk costing twelve cents would supply the body with about the same amount of nourishment as one pound of sirloin steak costing twenty-four cents.

Skim Milk, Cream and Butter.—The fatty part of milk is

32   FOOD FOR THE BODY

in the form of tiny balls which rise to the surface when milk is left standing several hours. This collection of fat balls or globules with the milk surrounding them is

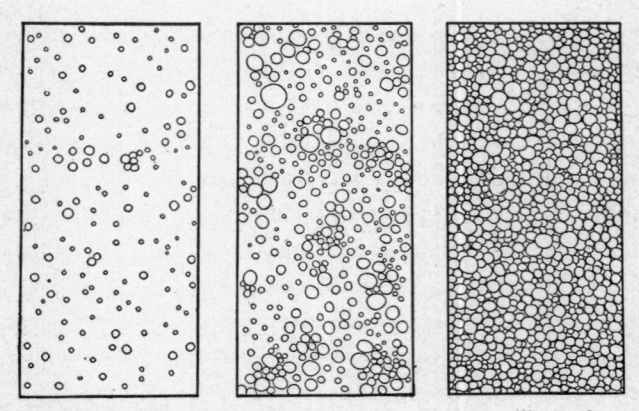

FIG. 21.—Tiny balls of fat in skim milk, whole milk and cream. Note how much more fat there is in cream.

called *cream*. When the cream is poured away or dipped off, the remaining bluish white fluid is known as *skim milk*.

By dashing the whole milk or only the cream about in a closed box or barrel, called a churn, the globules of fat are broken up and made to collect in yellow masses forming butter. It requires about three gallons of milk to make one pound of butter.

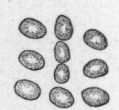

FIG. 22.—The bacteria which cause milk to sour. Much enlarged.

The milk from which the butter has been removed by churning is called *buttermilk*. It often has a sour taste due to the work of bacteria which changed the sugar of the sweet milk into an acid. Buttermilk is a healthful drink and aids digestion. Both buttermilk and skim milk are valuable foods. Two quarts of either of them will furnish nearly as much nourishment to the body as a pound of beef steak.

Soups.—Soups are made by placing vegetables or meats in cold water which is then gradually heated to near the boiling point. This temperature is maintained from a half hour to several hours, so as to dissolve out as much nourishment as possible from the solid parts.

Soups do not contain much nourishment but are useful at the beginning of a meal to start the flow of the digestive juices, and thus prepare for the real food to be eaten later. They also prevent one when very hungry from overeating, as they give the desired feeling of fulness without the presence of much solid matter.

Vegetable Foods.—Many vegetable foods contain a large amount of nourishment. Bread, corn meal, oatmeal, rice, potatoes, peas and beans have a large food value. They are also cheap foods and when well chewed are healthful. Ten cents' worth of oatmeal will yield more food for the body than forty cents' worth of beefsteak. Ten cents spent for small white dried beans will purchase more food for the body than fifty cents spent for smoked ham.

The common breakfast foods made from the cereals, wheat, corn, and oats, are healthful and nourishing, but more expensive than hominy, oatmeal or corn meal.

Turnips, cabbage, beets, lettuce and cauliflower, radishes, onions and asparagus contain much water and but little nourishment. They are useful in increasing the action of the digestive organs, and in supplying mineral matter. Their pleasing taste also gives a better appetite. Many headaches and other pains such as those from rheumatism may sometimes be avoided by refusing meats and using certain vegetables.

Fruits.—The fruits contain very little nourishment but furnish minerals and hasten the action of the digestive organs. Partly decayed or unripe fruit should never be used as it may cause serious sickness. Fruits may be eaten either raw or cooked. Before eating the larger fruits, the peel or outside skin which may bear bacteria and dirt should be removed.

Why Alcohol should not be used as Food.—Some scientists believe that alcohol, as found in beer or whisky, may be used by the body for food. Most scientific men, however, do not consider alcohol worthy of being called a food because it cannot be used day after day without hurting some of the organs in the body. In some cases it may furnish energy for work during a short period. It may also arouse and excite certain organs to do more work for a very short time, but soon these same organs, as a result of the unnatural urging, work much slower than usual.

Why Alcohol is not a complete Food.—Alcohol is not a complete food in any form, because it cannot build up muscle, blood, bone, or any other tissue in the body. A person fed plenty of alcohol and nothing else will starve to death.

Some persons think alcohol is a food because they do not feel hungry after taking a drink. It lessens the desire for real food only by deadening the nerves which tell of the true need of food. Ale and beer contain a little food because they have in them some sugar and other substances. The great chemist Liebig said: "Nine quarts of the best ale contain as much nourishment as would lie on the end of a table knife."

Practical Questions

1. Of what does the body consist? 2. Why does the body need food? 3. Name the two groups of foods. 4. In what foods does sugar occur? 5. Where is starch found? 6. In what food is fat present? 7. What is an oil? 8. Why is it harmful to eat more than the body needs? 9. What is dyspepsia? 10. Name some expensive foods. 11. Name some cheap foods. 12. What can you say of the use of meat? 13. Which cuts of meat are cheapest? 14. Tell what you know about the value of eggs for food. 15. Of what does milk consist? 16. What can you say of milk as a food? 17. Compare the value of milk with beefsteak. 18. How does skim milk differ from cream? 19. How is butter made? 20. How are soups made? 21. Of what use are soups? 22. What can you say of the value of vegetables for food? 23. How may headaches and rheumatism often be avoided? 24. Of what use are fruits? 25. Why should alcohol not be used as a food? 26. Why is alcohol not a complete food? 27. Why do some persons think alcohol is a food?

Suggestions for the Teacher

The teacher may impress upon the minds of the pupils the facts taught in this chapter by talking about the foods which they use at the different meals. In many cases the pupils will be found to be using foods giving too little real nourishment and to be spoiling the appetite by the frequent use of candies. The work in the school should be made a help in the home.

CHAPTER V

THE CARE AND COOKING OF FOOD

Preventing Waste.—In many households, a considerable amount of food is wasted because of poor cooking, or because it is allowed to spoil. Every house should be provided with a cool cellar or a refrigerator to prevent molds and bacteria from spoiling such food as meat, milk and cooked vegetables. Cold prevents largely the growth of such plants.

Much of the food remaining from a meal may, if kept cool, be fixed over into appetizing dishes for another day. Inquiries lately made among many families by the Government officers show that over one hundred million dollars worth of food is wasted annually in the United States.

Milk.—This requires more care than any other food. One of the chief causes of sickness and death among young children is bad milk. More than twice as many people die from dirty milk as from old age. Milk is made bad or sour by bacteria getting into it.

Milk drawn by clean hands into scalded tin or agate pails from clean cows kept in clean stables will contain very few bacteria. These will grow but little during the next three days, if the milk is cooled at once and placed in tight jars in a cold cellar or spring house. Milk should not be left in an open vessel as it absorbs odors and receives many bacteria always floating in the air.

How Milk May Cause Sickness.—Those who are sick or are just recovering from illness, should not handle milk, which is to be used by others. The bacteria which cause typhoid fever, scarlet fever, tonsilitis and diphtheria, grow very rapidly when they get into milk. Every year hundreds of people catch these diseases from using milk receiving bacteria from sick persons who have handled the milk. Any one who nurses the sick may carry disease germs from them to the milk vessels, or these may get the germs from being washed in impure water.

Cleaning Milk Vessels.—Many babies are killed every year by their own sisters or mothers who are careless in neglecting to clean properly the nursing bottle or other vessels. Cholera infantum and other similar sickness in babies usually results from unclean milk. A rubber tube must never be used in a nursing bottle because it cannot be cleaned. The *nursing bottle* and the nipple which slips over its wide mouth should be brushed thoroughly in cold water immediately after use. The bottle may then be washed with hot water and soap, and the nipple left until needed in a cup of water containing a pinch of sal soda. It must be rinsed before use.

Milk should always be delivered in sealed glass bottles, to prevent the entrance of dirt and bacteria which are blown about in the dusty streets when the milk is being handled. A vessel after being used for milk should be cleaned immediately by rinsing well in cold water and then washing in hot water with soap or washing soda. If possible, it should then be placed for a few minutes in boiling water or steam.

Preventing Sickness from Unclean Milk.—Sometimes it is necessary to use milk which is not known to come from healthy cows in a clean dairy. Children may get tuberculosis from the use of milk given by cows having this disease. It is therefore wise when there is a probability that the milk is impure to heat it very hot for twenty minutes without boiling it. This is called *pasteurizing* it. It is easily done by placing a jar or pan of milk into another larger pan of water which is kept steaming the required time. After heating, it should be quickly cooled and used within twenty-four hours. While being heated and cooled, the milk should be stirred to hasten the process.

Meats.—One should never use chicken or other meats which have been in cold storage for several weeks. *Canned meat* or any other meat which has an unpleasant odor is

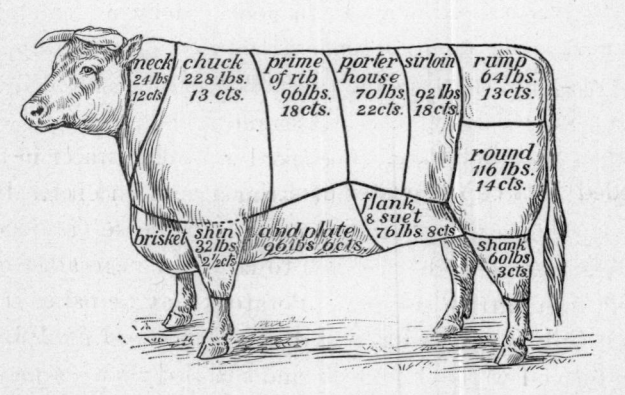

FIG. 23.—The names and prices of various cuts of beef.

likely to cause sickness because bacteria have grown in it and produced a poison. In warm weather, meat will remain good only one or two days in a cool cellar but if placed on ice it may be kept longer.

Roasted, broiled or stewed meats are more healthful than fried meats. Some cuts of meat are much more tender than others. Tender cuts such as round, sirloin and rump steaks and ribroast may be broiled or roasted. The tougher parts such as shoulder, chuck, brisket and belly, should be cooked in water in order to make them tender.

The water should be at the boiling point when the meat is placed in it so that the albumin of the outer part of the meat will be hardened and thus prevent the escape of the juices. After ten minutes' boiling, less heat should be used so that the water scarcely bubbles. This plan of cooking makes tough meat tender and nourishing.

Vegetables.—Potatoes, carrots, turnips, beets, onions, and cabbage may be kept in good condition for several weeks or even months in a cool cellar. Celery, tomatoes, and peas and beans in the pod will remain fresh only a day or two unless put in the refrigerator.

Most vegetables may be cooked in boiling water in from thirty to sixty minutes, but string beans and some beets often require three or four hours. To make the food as pleasing as possible, it is well to cook the vegetables often used, in a variety of ways. Potatoes may be baked in the oven with the skins on; pared, sliced raw and fried; boiled and served whole; or boiled and mashed with cream.

Vegetables purchased from the grocer in tin cans should

be removed from the cans as soon as they are opened to prevent the formation of poison from the tin.

Fruits.—With the exception of winter pears and apples, which will keep well several months in a cold room, most of the fruits spoil soon after being picked. Ripe berries and cherries will not remain good longer than one or two days after being gathered. The spoiling is always caused by molds or bacteria.

The careful housekeeper may preserve many of the fruits such as cherries, peaches, plums and berries by drying them several days in the sun or a few hours in the oven. Bacteria and mold need moisture for growth. These germs may also be prevented from growing by adding to the fruit an equal quantity of sugar while it is being cooked. Such food is known as *preserves*. Only a spoonful or two of such rich food should be eaten at one meal.

The best plan for *saving fruit* after cleaning it, is to place it in scalded glass jars with rubber rings and with the covers on loose. The germs are then killed by placing the jars in a hot oven a half hour, or more, after which they are tightly closed.

Planning the Meals.—One of the most important duties in the home is to provide the proper amount and kind of food for each meal. The list should always include foods that will form flesh and blood, and starch fats or sugars for fuel. A person fed only on fats, starches, and sugars, will starve because they do not make muscle and bone but give only heat and energy.

Bread, milk, lean meat, eggs, peas and beans are flesh-building foods. Potatoes, sugar, rice, corn and fat meat

THE CARE AND COOKING OF FOOD 41

will help the muscles do hard work and keep the body warm. People in cold weather like to eat fat meat because it keeps them warm.

Practical Questions

1. How may molds and bacteria be prevented from spoiling food? 2. What makes milk sour? 3. What care should be taken with milk? 4. Why should those just recovering from illness not handle milk to be used by other persons? 5. Describe how the baby's bottle should be cleaned. 6. How should any milk vessel be cleaned? 7. How is milk pasteurized? 8. What kind of milk should be pasteurized? 9. Why do canned meats sometimes cause sickness? 10. What is the most healthful way of cooking meats? 11. How may fruits be preserved? 12. For what two uses in the body should every meal furnish food? 13. Name the foods which would make a satisfying dinner at small cost. 14. Name some foods for breakfast which supply proper nourishment. 15. Why do we need more potatoes and fat meat in winter than in summer? 16. Why do bread and milk form a good supper?

Suggestions for the Teacher

The facts in this chapter may be emphasized by a valuable lesson in English in which each pupil is asked to describe how three or four of the common foods are cared for and cooked in the home. The information given by the pupils in their written papers will show that while some food is spoiled by improper care, much more is practically spoiled or made impalatable by the wrong method of cooking. Suggestions made in the class will often be put into practical use in the home.

CHAPTER VI

HOW FOOD IS USED BY THE BODY

The Organs of Digestion.—In order that food may support life, it must get into the blood and be carried to all parts of the body. It cannot enter the blood until it has been changed into a special souplike liquid. The process of making this liquid is called *digestion*. The organs used for this purpose form the *digestive system*. This consists of a tube over thirty feet long, called the *alimentary canal*, and other organs named *glands*.

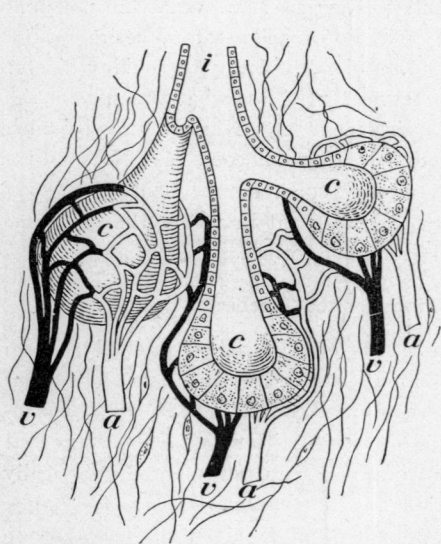

FIG. 24.—Diagram to show the working parts of a gland. *v* and *a* are blood tubes with thin-walled branches around the parts of the gland *c*. These take material from the blood and, after changing it, send it to the mouth, stomach or other places through the duct *i*.

Nature of a Gland.—A gland is a tiny straight or coiled tube or collection of branching tubes

HOW FOOD IS USED BY THE BODY

formed of cells (Fig. 24). A gland is able to take certain materials from the blood and manufacture them into a fluid useful to the body. The sweat moistening the skin and the fluid collecting in the mouth are formed by glands. The *liver* is the largest gland in the body and near to it is a small gland called the *pancreas*. The liquid formed by a gland is known as its *secretion*. The channel through which the secretion flows out is named the *duct*.

The Alimentary Canal.—The cavity within the trunk contains the greater part of the alimentary canal which is a tube for the digestion of the food. The trunk cavity is separated into two parts by a thin plate of tissue, known as the *diaphragm*.

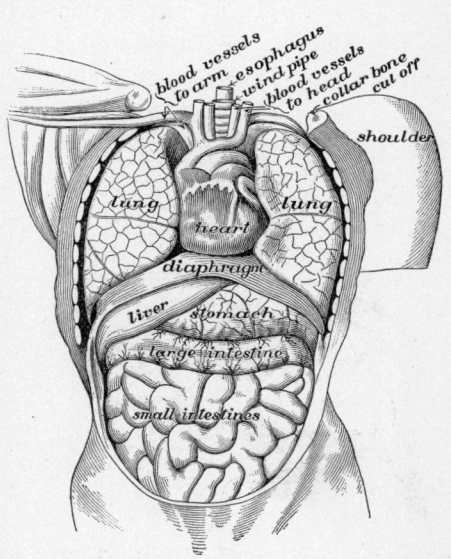

FIG. 25.—Organs in the body cavity viewed from the front.

The upper part, containing the heart, gullet and lungs, is the *cavity* of the *thorax*. The lower part, holding the stomach, intestines, liver, pancreas, spleen and other organs, is the *cavity* of the *abdomen*.

The alimentary canal consists of the *mouth*, *pharynx* or *throat*, *esophagus* or *gullet*, the *stomach* and *intestines*. The wall of the canal is made mostly of muscle, lined with a skinlike membrane which forms in addition to some digestive juices, a slippery fluid called *mucus*. This lining is therefore spoken of as *mucous membrane*.

Mucous membrane lines part of the cavity of the ear and nose, and all other channels in the body which the air touches. Mucus has the power to kill many harmful bacteria and it thus protects the body from disease.

Mouth Digestion.—The fluid which moistens the food in the mouth is called *saliva*. A quart of it is formed daily by three *salivary glands*. One of these glands lies below the ear, one is on the side of the tongue and another is under the tongue. Their secretion is brought to the mouth by ducts.

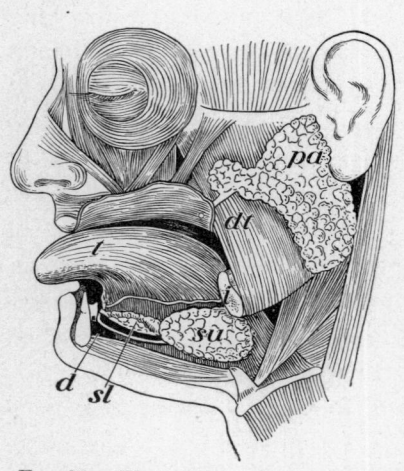

Fig. 26.—The salivary glands, *pa, su,* and *sl; t,* tongue; *d,* ducts opening into mouth.

The *chewing of food* causes the saliva to flow. The mixing of the food with the saliva increases the taste. The pleasing taste or odor of food makes the digestive juices flow into the stomach. The more food is chewed the better it will be digested in the stomach, because it will be in fine particles and there will be plenty of juice to act on them. Some of the starch of food is changed to sugar by the saliva. This is why dry bread tastes sweet after it has been chewed for some time.

Importance of Thorough Chewing.—Every mouthful of food should be chewed more than a dozen times. Experiments lately carried out prove that two thirds of a pound of food eaten, if well chewed, will furnish about the same nourishment to the body as a pound chewed in the usual way. More than a half hour is required to eat a meal properly. Foods like nuts and bananas, which are difficult to digest, may be digested by almost anyone who will take time to chew them thoroughly.

A very common cause of sickness known as *indigestion* or *dyspepsia* is swallowing food before it has been crushed into very fine particles. Headache and a pain in the region of the abdomen is usually the result of indigestion. Dizziness and even death may be due to imperfectly chewed food, which disturbs the action of the heart. To chew food thoroughly one should have good teeth.

Why Chewing Tobacco is Harmful.—When tobacco is chewed part of the poison in it is pressed out. This mixes with the juices in the mouth. The tender pink lining of the cheeks and tongue is full of tiny blood vessels. These drink in through their thin walls some of the tobacco poison and then it is carried by the blood tubes all over the body.

The poison of the tobacco is taken into the body very quickly. This is shown by the experience of boys when they use this harmful weed for the first time. A piece of tobacco as large as the thumb, if chewed only a few minutes by a boy not used to the poison, will make him dizzy and cause headache and other sick feeling. Some of the chapters which follow show how tobacco hurts a growing body. The chewing of tobacco also causes a great waste of saliva needed to help digest the food.

How Smoking Tobacco hurts the Mouth.—The smoke of the burning cigar or cigarette contains poison. This may be shown by drawing the smoke through water in which a fish is placed. In a short time the fish will die.

The blood vessels in the lining of the mouth take up some of the poison from the smoke. The blood then carries the poison to all parts of the body. Some of these are badly hurt by daily doses of poison.

The heat and gases from the burning tobacco numb the organs of taste in the tongue and other parts of the mouth. A smoker cannot then enjoy delicious food so much as one whose mouth is in perfect health.

How Alcoholic Drink affects the Mouth.—The organs of taste in the mouth are usually a safe guide in selecting food, but they may be injured by the use of alcohol. Few, if any, persons like beer or wine at first. These drinks, and also whisky and brandy, after daily use for several weeks, hurt the taste organs so that they are not satisfied with any other drink except that containing alcohol.

The strong desire for beer and wine is much more quickly aroused in the young than in those past middle life. On this account it is more dangerous for a boy to take a drink of liquor occasionally than it is for a man.

HOW FOOD IS USED BY THE BODY 47

The Teeth.—The mouth is furnished with two sets of teeth during life. The first set is known as *milk teeth*. There are ten of these in each jaw. The eight front ones used in biting off the food, are shaped like chisels and are called *incisors*. No teeth are present at birth, but all the incisors appear during the first year of life. The other milk teeth break through the gums by the time the child is two years of age. The eight back teeth of the milk set, used in crushing the food are the grinding teeth or *molars*.

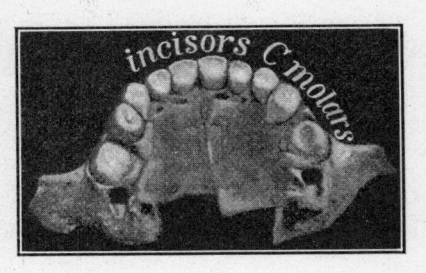

FIG. 27.—Teeth of the upper jaw at three years of age. *c* is the eye tooth.

Between the sixth and twelfth years, the roots of the milk teeth are absorbed, so that they drop out or may be easily pulled. The *permanent teeth* then grow into their places. In addition three permanent teeth appear in the back part of either half of each jaw. There are thirty-two perma-

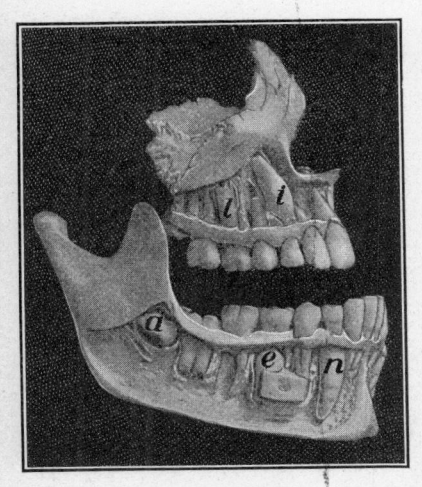

FIG. 28.—Part of the skull with the bone cut away to show permanent teeth *e* and *i* about to break through the gum.

48   HOW FOOD IS USED BY THE BODY

nent teeth. The first permanent molars appear at six years of age, just behind the milk teeth. The back tooth on each side in both jaws is commonly called the *wisdom* tooth. It appears between the eighteenth and twenty-fifth year of age.

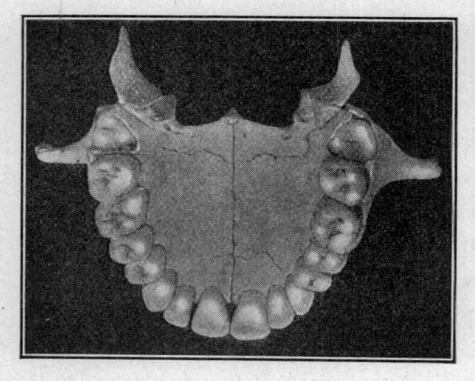

FIG. 29.—Teeth of a boy 18 years of age, in perfect condition. The wisdom tooth is just appearing.

Dogs, cats, horses and mice, all have two sets of teeth. Their teeth are shaped according to the work they have to do. The dog and cat, feeding on flesh, have sharp

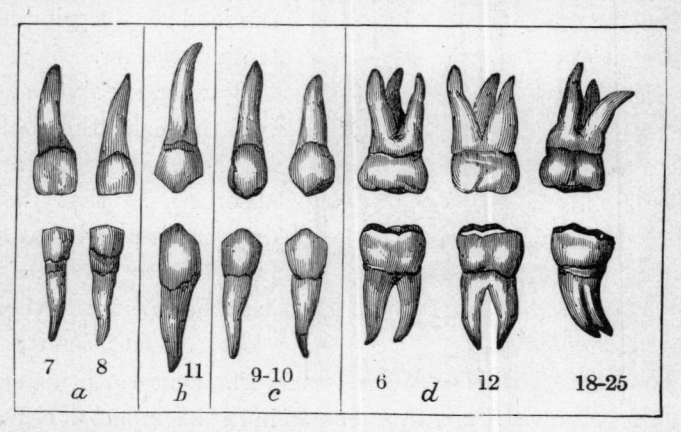

FIG. 30.—The permanent teeth of the right side. The numbers show at what age they appear; *a*, incisors; *b*, canines; *c*, premolars; *d*, molars.

HOW FOOD IS USED BY THE BODY

and cutting teeth, while the back teeth of the horse and cow have broad and flat grinding surfaces, to crush the hay and corn. Since man's back teeth are shaped for grinding and not for cutting such food as flesh, we ought to use much vegetable food.

How the Teeth may be Ruined.—The outer part of the tooth is covered with a thin layer of hard shiny substance called *enamel*. This protects the inner bony part or *dentine* from bacteria which cause decay. Bits of sweets, or other food particles, clinging to the teeth after eating, make the bacteria grow rapidly and produce an acid. This may soften the enamel and thus let the acid and bacteria get to the bony part of the tooth, which then decays rapidly. For this reason a strong thread called dental floss, or a tooth pick of quill, or of wood, should be used to remove the bits of food from between the teeth after eating.

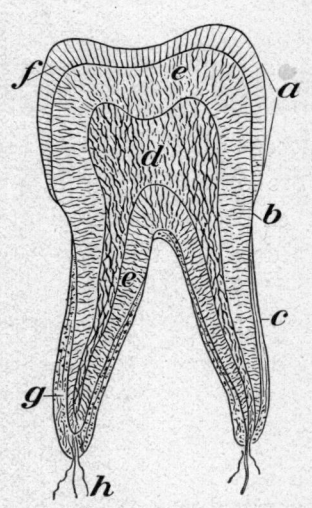

FIG. 31.—Section through a tooth. *a*, crown; *b*, neck; *c*, root; *d*, pulp of nerves and blood tubes; *e*, dentine; *f*, enamel; *g*, cement; *h*, nerves and vessels.

The Care of the Teeth.—A *tooth brush* and warm water should be used morning and night to clean thoroughly, both the inner and outer surfaces of the teeth. To clean the upper teeth the brush should be drawn from the gum downward. To clean the lower teeth the brush should be drawn from the gum upward. A little good tooth powder used on the brush once a day is helpful.

The *care of the teeth* in childhood will prevent much pain and sickness in later years. The cracking of nuts, or the biting off of thread or the ends of the finger nails is hurtful to teeth, as the enamel is likely to be cracked. The teeth should be examined twice a year by a dentist, and any decayed places repaired. Even the milk teeth often need to be repaired. Decaying teeth make the mouth sore so that the food is not well chewed. The stomach may then become sick and other illness follow. The cavities in decaying teeth are breeding places for disease germs.

Stomach Digestion.—After the food has been chewed it passes back to the *pharynx* and is then squeezed into the gullet named *esophagus*. This is a straight tube leading from the throat to the stomach.

The stomach is a half-gallon sac, with an outer wall of muscle lined within by mucous membrane, made largely of *gastric glands* of which there are more than a million. These glands, each consisting

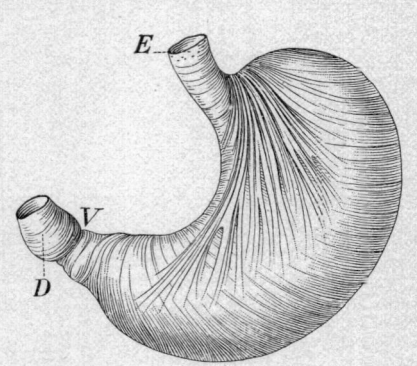

FIG. 32.—The stomach showing the muscles which churn the food. *E*, where food enters; *V*, entrance into the intestine, *D*.

of a tube with several branches, give out daily three quarts of *gastric juice* to dissolve the lean meat and other like foods.

Gastric Juice.—The gastric juice is made to mix with the food by the action of the stomach muscles, which squeeze the contents back and forth. If the stomach is too full, there is no room for the food to move about

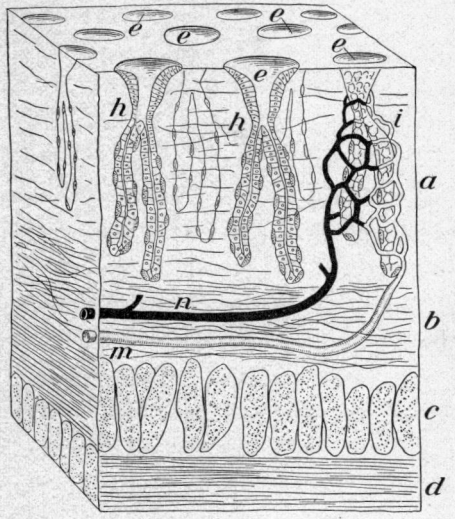

FIG. 33.—A tiny block out of the stomach wall. *a*, the mucous membrane; *c* and *d*, the muscles; *h*, gastric glands; *m* and *n*, blood tubes to the glands; *e*, mouth of glands within the stomach.

and mix with the juices. Sickness called indigestion may be the result. The quickest relief is given by vomiting.

Some persons do not have enough gastric juice to digest even a small quantity of food. They can nearly double the flow of gastric juice by chewing the food twice as long as usual. Funny stories and pleasant experiences related at meal time also help digestion.

After remaining in the stomach from one to five hours, the food is like thick gravy and is called *chyme*. It is then pushed in small quantities through the gateway formed by a circular muscle, into the intestine.

The Intestines.—The *small intestine* receives the food from the stomach. It is a coiled tube about twenty feet long (Fig. 34). It fills up much of the abdominal cavity and is held in place by a thin glistening membrane attached to the region of the backbone. The wall of the intestine is like that of the stomach. The outer part is of muscle and the lining is mucous membrane made largely of tiny, tubelike

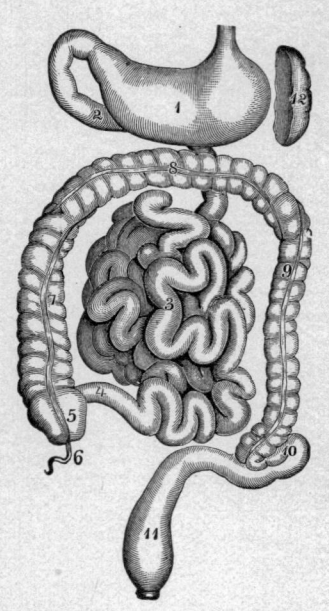

Fig. 34.—The stomach and intestines; 1, stomach; 5, 7, 8, 9, 10, 11, large intestine; 3, small intestine; 4, entrance of small intestine into large one; 12, spleen.

glands. The mucous membrane is much wrinkled into cross folds, while over its whole surface stick out millions of tiny fingerlike projections called *villi* (Fig. 36).

A few inches below the stomach, ducts from the pancreas and liver empty into the intestine. The

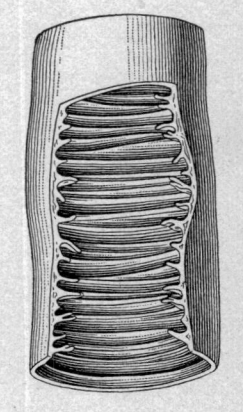

Fig. 35.—Piece of small intestine cut open to show wrinkling of inner coat bearing villi.

secretion of the pancreas is *pancreatic juice*, and that of the liver is *bile*.

The *large intestine* receives the waste part of the food from the small intestine, and retains it a few hours until some of the water is absorbed. This waste matter should be expelled from the body at about the same time each day. Neglecting to do this, often causes serious illness.

Intestinal Digestion.—The liquid food is kept moving in the small intestine by the movement of its muscular walls. In this way the food is well mixed with the bile and pancreatic juice, and also the other juice formed by the intestinal glands. The food is acted on

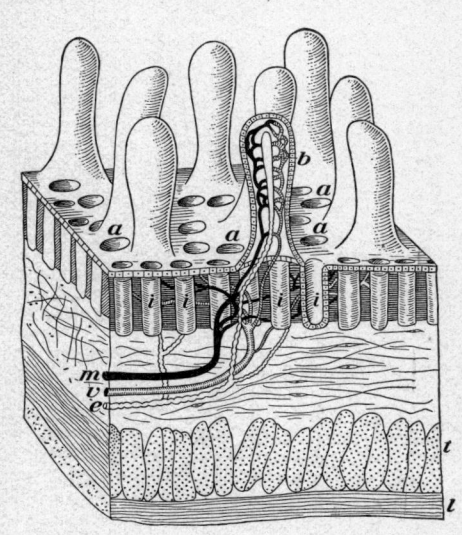

Fig. 36.—A tiny block cut from the wall of the intestine showing villi and the mouths of glands at *a*; *b*, villus cut open to show the lacteal *e* and blood tubes *m* for absorbing food.

and changed by these several juices into a dark fluid called *chyle*. It is then ready to be received by the blood vessels, and carried to the heart, toes, fingers and other parts of the body.

Nearly all the nourishment received by the body is taken from the food while in the small intestine. The waste or unused portion of the food, with some of the bile, then passes on into the large intestine, from which it should be expelled once each day to avoid the collection of too much poisonous refuse causing a sluggish action of the bowels called *constipation*.

The best means of *preventing constipation* is by exercise, the drinking of much water, especially in the morning before breakfast, and the eating of fruits.

How the Food enters the Blood.—The chyle of the intestine is so watery that it will pass through the thin membrane lining the intestine. The cells forming the membrane help the passage or absorption of the food. The membrane is full of tiny blood tubes, with walls much thinner than tissue paper, so that the watery food can get through them. The absorbing surface is much increased by the cross folds of the membrane, and the millions

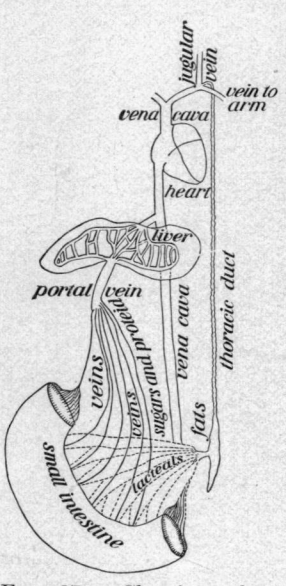

FIG. 37. — Showing how food goes from the intestines into the blood.

of tiny outgrowths, the *villi*. These contain networks of blood tubes to receive the food. It is then carried to the liver. From here it goes to the large vein entering the heart, which sends it with the blood throughout the body.

In the center of each villus is another kind of tube called

a lacteal, because it takes up the milky or fatty parts of the food. This lacteal unites with thousands of similar lacteals from other villi, to carry their food to a duct passing up along the backbone to enter a blood tube in the neck. Since the villi take up most of the food they are called *absorbents*. A little food and considerable alcohol may be absorbed by the blood tubes in the wall of the stomach.

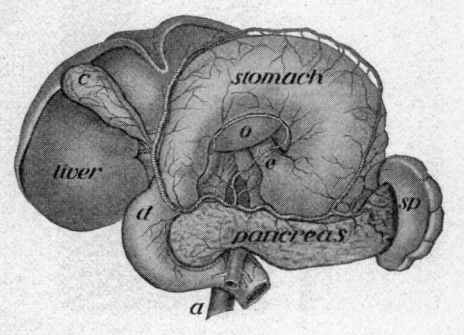

FIG. 38.—The stomach pulled upward to show the pancreas; *d*, intestine; *sp*, spleen; *c*, gall bladder.

Pancreas and Liver.—The *pancreas*, called by the butchers *sweetbreads*, is a long, flat, pinkish gland, just back of the stomach (Fig. 38). It sends about a quart of juice into the intestine daily. This is the most important of all the digestive juices, because it acts on all kinds of food, and prepares them to enter the blood.

The *liver* is the largest gland of the body. It is of a dark red color, and lies directly below the diaphragm. On its under side is a sac, called the *gall bladder*, used in storing bile when there is no food in the intestine.

The chief *use of the liver*, besides forming bile and stopping many of the poisons that may enter the body with the food, is to change sugars into a kind of starch, and store it until needed. It also changes some of the waste matter of the body into a form so that it can pass out through the kidneys, when carried there by the blood.

Eating and Health.— In young persons, most of the headache, feverishness, foul breath, and pain in the stomach and intestines result from not giving the digestive organs the right kind of care. Children often eat too much candy, pickles and rich food, and wash their food down with a swallow of water, instead of chewing

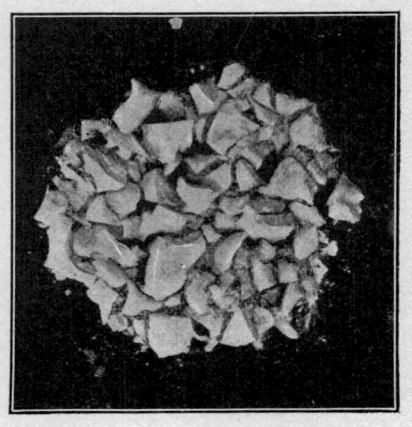

FIG. 39.—Hard boiled white of egg chewed ten times.

it enough to break it into fine bits and moisten it completely with saliva.

After six years of age children should eat only three times daily. The taking of food every two or three hours spoils the appetite, and makes the organs give out a weaker digestive juice. Cake, candy and pies or preserves should be

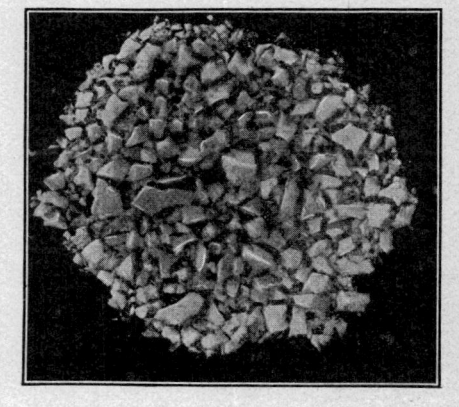

FIG. 39.—Hard boiled white of egg chewed fifty times.

eaten only at meal time, and then in small quantities. Sweetmeats often tempt persons to eat too much, and therefore plain food is much better for children. Some foods such as cucumbers, raw onions and hot bread are hard to digest, and should be used very sparingly by children.

Digestion is greatly aided by fresh air and exercise, but violent exercise should not be taken within an hour after eating, as it draws the blood away from the stomach where it is needed to form gastric juice. The use of alcoholic drinks, or much tea, coffee, or ice water at meal time is a common cause of indigestion.

How Strong Drink hurts the Stomach.—The soft, tender lining of the stomach is full of blood vessels forming a rich network. Strong drink, even in small quantities, makes these vessels become larger. This causes the glands to pour out gastric juice when it is not needed. In those taking strong wine or whisky several times daily, the vessels of the stomach remain constantly enlarged. The natural pink color of the stomach lining becomes changed to a reddish hue like the mucous lining of the throat when it is sore.

Alcohol may also cause certain glands in the stomach to pour out a thick, slimy fluid, like that in the nose during a cold. This ropy mucus surrounds the particles of food so that the digestive juices cannot dissolve them.

Wine and Whisky hinder Digestion.—Some doctors think that a little wine taken at meal time by older persons helps digestion. Late experiments show that wine and whisky help digestion but little in any case, and in some persons they make digestion slower.

Alcohol weakens the action of the muscles in the walls of the stomach, so that they do not squeeze the food about and mix it with the gastric juice. The food may lie in a mass while germs of decay act on it, and thus cause bad breath.

The cause of improvement in many delicate persons, after giving up the use of beer and wine, is often due to better digestion brought about by the strong action of the stomach muscles.

Learning how Alcohol affects the Stomach.—Wine sometimes makes persons feel better after taking it with their meals because it numbs the nerves which would otherwise tell of any pain in the stomach. The real effect of strong drink on digestion has been learned by studying people who have used alcohol for a time and then lived without it.

A man by the name of St. Martin had a hole shot through the front wall of his body, and into his stomach. As the wound healed leaving an opening, the doctors were able to watch the digestion of the food, and the effects of the alcohol given him. Much alcohol caused blood to ooze out from the tender lining of the stomach.

Practical Questions

1. How is food changed before it enters the blood? 2. What is a gland? 3. Name some glands. 4. What is a duct? 5. What is the alimentary canal? 6. What are the two parts of the trunk cavity? 7. Name the chief organs in each. 8. Where is mucous

HOW FOOD IS USED BY THE BODY

membrane present? 9. What forms the saliva? 10. What is the result of chewing food? 11. Why should food be chewed thoroughly? 12. Why is chewing tobacco harmful? 13. In what way does smoking injure the mouth? 14. How does alcohol affect the mouth? 15. Describe the milk teeth. 16. When does the first permanent tooth appear? 17. How many permanent teeth are there? 18. Describe the enamel. 19. What causes teeth to decay? 20. Why should the teeth be brushed often? 21. How many decaying teeth have you? 22. Describe the stomach. 23. How is the food mixed with the juices of the stomach? 24. How can the quantity of gastric juice be increased? 25. Describe the small intestine. 26. Tell how the food is changed in the small intestine. 27. How does the food get into the blood? 28. Describe the pancreas. 29. Describe the liver. 30. How does alcohol affect the stomach?

Suggestions for the Teacher

During the study of this chapter, the teacher should observe the teeth of the pupils and where necessary, by a kind note to the parents suggest the importance of preserving the teeth as an aid to health. Among the lower grades nearly four fifths of the pupils are found to have decayed teeth which in many cases will later cause serious sickness and in some instances death.

CHAPTER VII

DRINK AND HEALTH

Use of Water.—Most people do not drink so much water during cold weather as the body needs. The body requires about three quarts of water daily to supply the wants of the tissues and wash the impurities out of the system. Since not much more than a quart of water is present in the daily amount of food used, at least six glasses of water should be drunk.

The use of much *ice water* is unhealthy, and may cause sickness when one is very warm. Some people injure their health by trying to satisfy their thirst with beer or whisky. Pure, cool, water is the best liquid to quench the thirst.

Impure Water.—More than a hundred thousand persons in this country are made ill every year, by the use of impure water. Three fourths of all cases of typhoid fever come from the use of water containing the germs of this disease.

Nearly all rivers supplying water to cities and towns contain some typhoid germs. Through the carelessness of the sick, or those who care for them, the germs may get into springs and wells. Water which looks clear may be very dangerous. The water of a stream running through an inhabited region is not safe to drink without special treatment.

How Water is made Unsafe.—Meat and other foods are spoiled by many kinds of bacteria. Water may have thousands of bacteria in every cupful, but it will cause no disease, unless the germs from sick persons, or animals, are present. The green plants often seen growing in springs do not harm the water.

A well near a barnyard or cesspool is likely to be unsafe for use. The liquids enter the soil, and sometimes follow

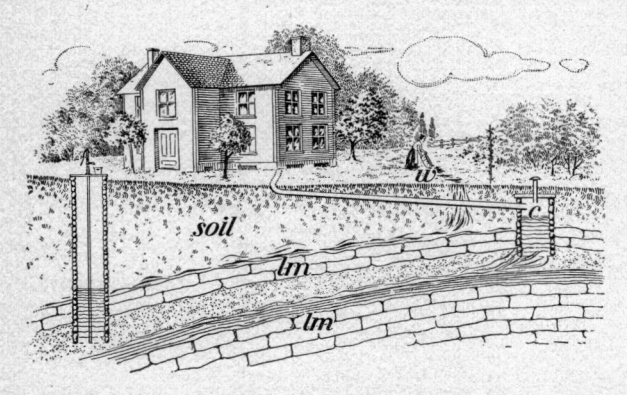

FIG. 40.—How the well often becomes impure and carries disease.

along the crevice in rocks a hundred feet or more. *Sewage*, which is household waste, *garbage*, or dead animals cast into a stream, or placed near a well or spring, may cause many deaths among those using the water. The excretions from one person sick with typhoid fever, near Wilkesbarre, in Pennsylvania, were thrown out on the bank of a stream, and caused over a thousand cases of fever, and more than one hundred deaths among those using the water, several miles down the stream.

How to make Water Safe.—Any water may be made

safe for drinking by boiling it one minute. Longer boiling gives the water a flat taste. The water may be cooled over night in a stone jar, and then placed in the ice box.

Many of the cities run their water through a layer of sand and stones to remove the germs. This is known as *filtration* or *filtering* of the water. Any city using river water may save much sickness, and many lives yearly, by filtering the drinking water. During the years 1900 to 1905, thousands of people in Pittsburg, New Orleans and Philadelphia died from the use of impure water.

The Alcoholic Drinks.—The alcoholic drinks, often called liquors or strong drinks, are composed largely of water, alcohol, and flavors. None of these drinks contain any disease germs, but when used day after day they often cause weakness, and disease in some organs of the body. The common drinks containing alcohol are: *whisky, beer, brandy, rum, wine, porter, ale, cider,* and *birch beer.*

Why Alcoholic Drinks are used.—Some people drink whisky in cold weather because they think it makes them warm, and others use it in warm weather to make them cool. As alcohol partially deadens the feelings, the drinker does not know when he is hot or cold.

When persons feel lazy and dull they sometimes take a drink, to make them feel lively and cheerful. As this pleasant effect of a drink lasts only an hour or two, more drink must be taken frequently. In this way an unnatural thirst is developed, and one feels a continual longing for liquor. If he continues to satisfy the longing day after day, an awful appetite is likely to grow in him, until he is no longer able to keep from drinking, even though he may try very hard.

Some persons drink to forget sorrow and trouble. It is very foolish to do this, because the effect of the drink wears off in a few hours, and then the sorrow is more bitter than ever. Others drink to be social, and because for a short time the drink helps them to talk more glibly. Drinking for such reasons is unwise, because alcohol puts their common sense to sleep and they are likely to do and say very foolish things.

How Alcohol is made.—Alcohol is made by the growth of yeast in some liquid containing sugar. Yeast is a tiny plant having somewhat the shape of a football. The yeast cake bought at the store contains millions of these plants. They may be easily seen in a bit of yeast cake, mashed up in a drop of water, under the microscope. Warmth causes the plants to grow and change part of the sugar to alcohol and carbon dioxide.

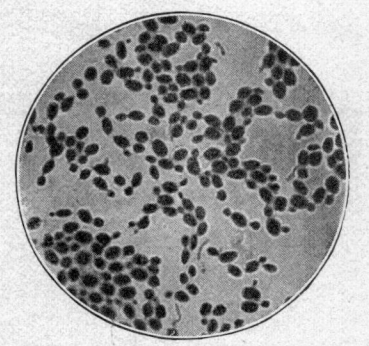

If a part of a yeast cake is put in a glass of sweetened water kept warm, a bubbling or frothing of the liquid will occur in two or three hours. The action produced by the growing yeast is called *fermentation*. Alcohol is then formed as may be learned by the biting or sour taste of the liquid.

Fig. 41.—Yeast plants used in making beer. Much enlarged.

Beer.—Beer, ale and porter are called *malt liquors*. They are so named from the *malt* used in making them. Malt is grain, sprouted to change its starch into sugar. Barley is the grain used in making beer. The yeast plant uses the sugar of the barley to make the alcohol. Hops are added to give the proper flavor to the beer.

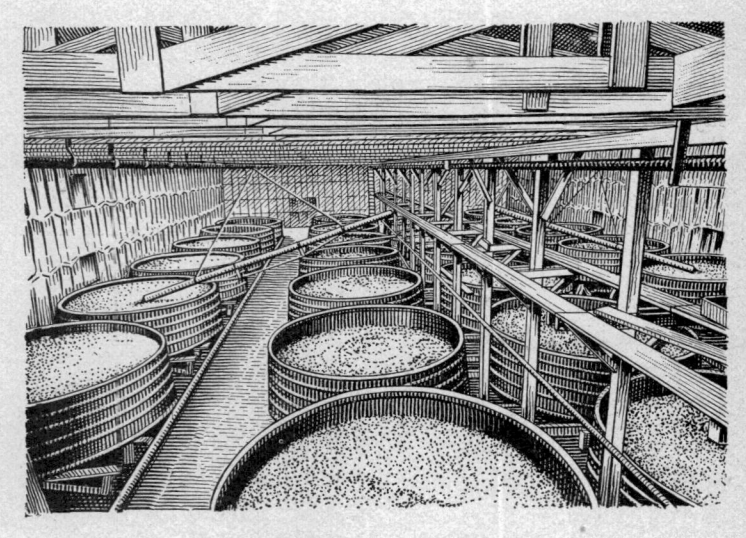

FIG. 42.—Vats in a wine room for fermentation.

Beer contains but little alcohol, and is not useful for food as it contains but a trifle of nourishment. It may help one who eats plenty of food to get fat, because it prevents the oxidation of those substances which form fat in the body. This kind of fat is not a sign of health.

Wine.—Wine is called a *fermented* liquor because it is produced by a fermentation of the juice of such fruits as

DRINK AND HEALTH 65

grapes, berries and cherries. The fermentation is brought about by the wild yeast, commonly present on the surface of fruit. Sugar for the growth of the yeast is in the fruit. Most wine is made from grapes. It usually contains from ten to twenty parts of alcohol. *Claret* and *champagne* are weak wines.

In making wine, the grapes are thrown into a large wooden tub. They must then be crushed to make the juice run out. This is sometimes done by men, who walk around on the grapes in bare feet. After this mass has fermented several days the juice is drawn off in bottles.

Whisky and Brandy.—These are the strongest of alcoholic drinks. They are about one half pure alcohol. As the yeast plants cannot continue to grow in a solution after one seventh part of it is alcohol, the stronger drinks are made from the weaker solutions by a process called *distillation*.

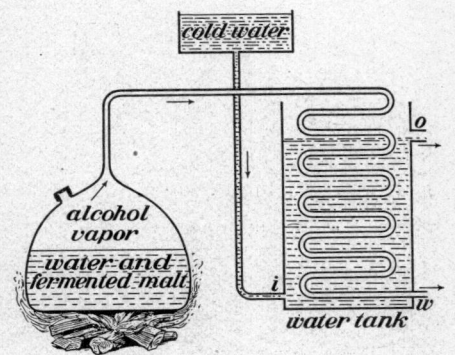

FIG. 43.—Simple still for distillation of whisky. *w*, the outlet for the whisky.

Heat changes alcohol into a vapor or steam much quicker than it does water. When the fermented solution containing alcohol and water is heated, the alcohol vapor passes off and is collected and cooled, so as to become a liquid again. This is distillation. In this way whisky is made from corn, rye and barley. Brandy is made from fermented fruit juice in a similar manner.

Patent Medicines.—Many of the liquid patent medicines contain more alcohol than is present in beer, and some of them are so strong in alcohol that two or three tablespoonfuls would make a child drunk. Many people have been known to get drunk by using patent medicines, which have fixed on them the terrible alcoholic thirst.

Patent medicines which contain alcohol and other

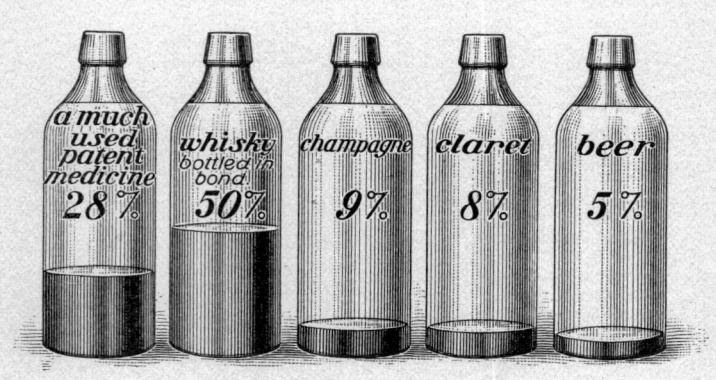

FIG. 44.—The amount of alcohol in various drinks.

harmful drugs should not be used. The good results, which they occasionally seem to give, is generally due to some stimulant, or to some sleep-producing drugs, which later cause harm. Thousands of lives have been wrecked, and others shortened, by using patent medicines, instead of consulting a physician. Any medicine advertised as a sure cure for several ailments should be regarded as worthless.

Cider.—Some persons who never take other alcoholic

drinks use a considerable quantity of cider, without realizing that it contains alcohol. The wild yeast plants, present nearly everywhere, get into the cider when the juice is pressed out of the apples. The yeast will grow so rapidly, that after three days of warm weather, the cider may contain more alcohol than is present in beer. Cider in this condition has a sour and *biting taste*, and is said to be hard. Two or three glasses of very *hard cider* are likely to make one drunk. Soon after the cider becomes hard, certain bacteria change the alcohol into vinegar.

Soft Drinks.—*Soda water*, *ginger ale*, *lemon soda* and other similar beverages are called soft drinks, because they contain no alcohol. The *biting taste* is due to carbon dioxide, with which they are charged. They are healthful when used in moderation. Birch beer is not strictly a soft drink, because it contains about one third as much alcohol as other beer.

Alcohol Injures the Health.—A few years ago there was organized a committee, composed of fifty business men and scientists, to investigate the results of using beer, wine and whisky. Through careful inquiries, from hundreds of people in different states, they learned that about 1,000,000 men in our country are every year drinking to such excess as to injure their health.

Very few, if any, persons can drink liquor daily for many years, without causing disease in some of the organs. The use of much alcohol often produces disease in the liver, kidneys, heart or other blood vessels, and does lasting injury to the nervous system.

The records of one of the large insurance companies

show that those persons not using alcoholic drinks suffer but little over one half as many weeks sickness as the drinkers. Experiments show that alcohol weakens the system, and makes it an easy prey to disease caused by bacteria.

Alcohol makes Persons Weak.—It was once thought that the use of wine and whisky gave strength. Many observations and experiments, lately made, show that they really weaken both mind and body. Actual tests prove that those who use alcoholic beverages cannot lift so heavy a weight, run so fast, or shoot so straight as the total abstainers.

Careful records show that such diseases as pneumonia and tuberculosis are more likely to attack habitual drinkers than those whose bodies are not weakened by alcohol. The persons soonest overcome with cold in winter, and heat in summer are the beer drinkers, and lovers of wine and whisky.

Alcohol makes People Poor.—The one great agent making people homeless and hungry, is strong drink. Records tell in accurate figures, that more than one third of the thousands of poor, living in the almshouses of this country, were brought there by the use of alcoholic drinks.

Inquiry into the cause of the condition of over five thousand homeless children, brought forth the information that over two thousand of them owed their sad state to the use of alcoholic drink by the parents. The habitual drinker not only spends much money for his destroying drink, but renders himself unfit to perform any careful work to earn money.

Alcohol makes People Wicked.—Strong drink often ruins not only the body, but also the character. Many persons who are honest when sober, have been led to steal, and even murder, while under the influence of liquor. Alcohol weakens the will, and lets the evil nature control the man.

Inquiry concerning thirteen hundred convicts in our state prisons and reformatories a few years ago, led to the discovery that alcoholic drink caused a large proportion of these criminals to be guilty of crime. In some of the counties of certain states where the law does not allow the sale of liquor, the jail is empty much of the time.

Danger in using Alcoholic Drinks.—Some persons can take strong drink occasionally without injuring their health. They may, however, do much harm by leading others to drink, who little by little fasten on themselves the destroying appetite.

A young person who drinks occasionally is much more likely to become intemperate than a person over fifty years of age, because alcohol has a greater effect on the nervous system of the young than the aged. About one in every ten occasional drinkers becomes a drunkard. The habitual use of alcoholic drinks for a few years in youth is almost certain to so weaken the will and to poison the tissues that the user cannot quit drinking without taking special treatment to cure his sick body.

Quick Effect of Alcohol.—Alcohol was once thought to be a stimulant. A *stimulant* is anything which causes the organs of the body to work faster. Alcohol is now called a *narcotic*. This is any drug which tends to produce sleepiness and dull pain. A small amount of whisky may cause some of the organs to work more quickly for a few minutes, but for a much longer time it makes the same organs work slower than usual.

Practical Questions

1. Why should we drink much water? 2. What is the danger from impure water? 3. How is water made unsafe? 4. How may any water be made safe for drinking? 5. Does filtering water prevent sickness? 6. Name some drinks containing alcohol. 7. Why do some persons drink liquor? 8. Why is it unwise to use alcoholic drinks? 9. Describe how alcohol is made. 10. What are malt liquors? 11. Describe how wine is made. 12. Describe distillation. 13. Why should persons not use patent medicines? 14. Give facts showing that alcohol injures health. 15. What shows that alcohol makes people weak? 16. State facts showing that alcohol makes people poor. 17. How is it known that alcohol makes persons wicked? 18. What is the danger in using alcoholic drink? 19. What is a stimulant? 20. What is a narcotic?

Suggestions for the Teacher

The fact that a quarter million of our people have died within the last ten years from the use of impure water shows that it is worth while for the teacher to make special inquiries from the pupils as to the source of their drinking water. A brief discussion of the subject may lead to a remedy for the use of unclean cisterns and doubtful wells which will prevent unnecessary sickness and death in the future.

CHAPTER VIII

TOBACCO AND OTHER NARCOTICS AND THEIR EFFECT ON HEALTH

Nature of Narcotics.—A narcotic is that which when taken into the body tends to deaden pain, produce sleepiness, and make some of the organs act more slowly. Alcohol, tobacco, laudanum and many patent medicines are common narcotics.

In the beginning, the taste of narcotics is often unpleasant, and may make the user sick. By daily use his system becomes accustomed to the poison until he is compelled to take large quantities to satisfy the unnatural appetite.

How Tobacco is made.—Tobacco is the dried and cured leaves of a plant growing to the height of three or four feet. The states raising the largest amount of tobacco are Kentucky, North Carolina, Virginia, Tennessee and Ohio.

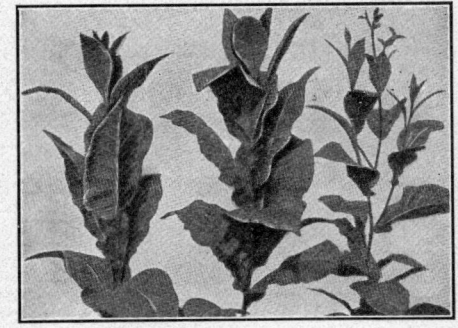

FIG. 45.—Tobacco plants.

Chewing tobacco is made by pressing the leaves into the

form of blocks which are cut into fine shreds. In the manufacture of *cigars*, some of the leaves are formed into a roll and then a piece of a large leaf is wrapped around it.

A *cigarette* is a small roll of tobacco usually held together by a paper wrapper. Some smokers make their own cigarettes from fine-cut tobacco.

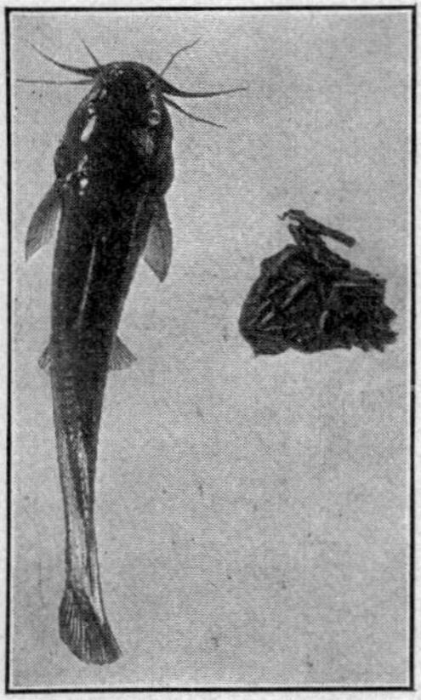

Fig. 46.—This fish was killed in twenty-five minutes by the poison soaked out of the bunch of tobacco at the right and placed in an aquarium with the fish.

Poison from Tobacco.—Many persons after the age of twenty years use tobacco all their lives and seem not to be harmed by it. It is likely, however, that in numerous cases some of the organs are prevented from doing their best work. In the young who use much tobacco, certain organs are seriously weakened by the poison. This poison is *nicotine*.

If a pipeful of tobacco be boiled in a cup of water much of the poison will be drawn out into the water. If this poisoned water is then put into a quart jar of water containing a small fish, it will kill the fish in less than a half hour.

Harm in Smoking.—Some people think they can smoke without any bad results, because they believe the burning of the tobacco will destroy the poison. This is not true. The nicotine is drawn into the mouth with the smoke, and is then absorbed into the blood. The burning of the tobacco also gives rise to another poison.

The smoking of cigars, or of tobacco in a pipe, is less harmful than using cigarettes. The smoking of tobacco, in any form by young persons, prevents proper growth, by making the cells act too slowly, and thus neglect doing their whole duty. It lessens the sense of taste, sometimes causes a poor appetite, and in other ways has an unwholesome effect on the organs of digestion. Some schools, realizing how the health may be injured by tobacco, have absolutely prohibited its use among their pupils.

Cigarettes.—The cigarette habit is dangerous to young people. The small cost of a single smoke and the mildness of the tobacco tempt boys to form a habit which very few are strong enough to break away from, even when they learn it will gradually weaken the body. Serious sickness, insanity and death have resulted from excessive cigarette smoking. It is so harmful to boys that many business men will not employ those accustomed to use cigarettes.

It is the duty of states to make such laws as will protect health and prevent crime. Some states have, therefore, passed laws preventing the sale and manufacture of cigarettes within their borders. Since 1896, when people learned the danger from the use of cigarettes, the number manufactured in the United States has decreased about one half.

The Chewing of Tobacco.—The chewing of tobacco is an uncleanly habit, as well as injurious to health. It causes a great waste of saliva which is much needed to act on the food. Using tobacco in this way permits so much poison to enter the system that it sometimes affects the heart.

To get rid of some of the poison, the tobacco chewer

must constantly indulge in the unclean habit of spitting. This makes him disagreeable to others and prevents him from securing employment with many business houses.

Snuff.—Snuff is tobacco ground into a fine powder to which other materials are sometimes added. Snuff using was a common habit among both men and women a hundred years ago, but it has long been out of style. The snuff was drawn up the nose so as to affect the delicate nerve endings, and cause the person to sneeze. Snuff tends to cause soreness in the nose and throat.

Opium.—Opium, like tobacco, is used by thousands of people for the pleasant effect it produces. The drug is made from the white poppy, grown in Asia Minor, Egypt, India, Persia and China. By cutting gashes in the head of the poppy, a fluid is made to run out and form a gummy substance. From this the pure opium is secured.

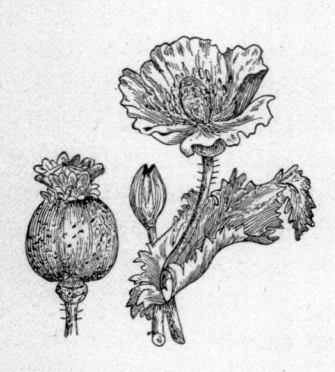

FIG. 47.—The opium plant.

Use of Opium.—Opium is much used in medicine to produce sleep, numb pain, and quiet the organs of the body. Opium forms the most important part of paregoric, laudanum and most soothing sirups. *Morphine* is a strong form of opium. Opium and morphine are dangerous drugs, and should not be used, except by the advice of a physician.

In China, and in some other countries, opium is smoked

and also eaten by persons who have acquired the habit, and are unable to stop it. In this way it has ruined the body, mind and character of thousands of people. Laws have been made to stop its use in some countries. Japan no longer allows it to be sold, except for medicine.

Danger in Using Drugs.—No one can form the habit of using opium or morphine, without making himself miserable, and injuring his health very much. The use of these drugs regularly, for only one month, will, in many cases, fix the habit so firmly on a person that he cannot stop it without help. Nearly one million persons are suffering from the opium or morphine habit in the United States.

The many advertisements in newspapers and magazines, offering to cure the opium or morphine habit, are by dishonest persons who rob drug victims of thousands of dollars yearly. A physician at home should be asked to direct the cure of the patient. *Cocaine* is another dangerous drug, which should not be used except by the advice of a physician.

How the Drug Habit is brought on.—No one expects to become a slave to any drug when he begins using it. Some persons take a drug to make them sleep, and others to soothe pain or help a headache. The dose, from week to week, must be constantly increased to produce the desired effect, because the system becomes accustomed to the poison. Before the user is aware of it, the terrible drug habit fixes itself on him, and he finds himself in a nervous state of unrest, which nothing helps except another dose of the drug.

Laudanum, Paregoric and Soothing Sirups.—Many people

have acquired the drug habit by using laudanum, which contains much opium. Paregoric is a mixture of alcohol and other drugs, with a small amount of opium. Soothing sirups wrongly given to babies, to stop them from crying and produce sleep, contain some form of opium.

Cough medicines very often have in them opium, morphine or chloroform. None of these drugs should be used, as they weaken the body and injure the health, and are likely to cause a false appetite leading the victim to ruin.

Patent Medicines.—A patent medicine is a drug mixture which is advertised to cure one or several diseases, and whose contents are supposed to be unknown to all except the manufacturer. A reliable physician knows the value of all drugs used in patent medicines, and can select the one which is best suited to help each special ailment.

Many patent medicines are advertised to cure consumption. None of them, except codliver oil preparations, help the disease, and most of them make it worse. The few who say that patent medicines have helped them are likely mistaken, as most sick persons get well without medicine.

Danger in Using Patent Medicines.—Every year the people of our country pay $75,000,000 for patent medicines. Some of them make persons drunkards, some make their users slaves to the opium habit, and others cause death. Nearly all liquid patent medicines contain alcohol. The advertised cures for cold, coughs and consumption often contain chloroform, morphine, strychnine and other poisons. Cocaine is generally present in remedies offered to cure catarrh. Headache powders have caused a number of sudden deaths, due to a powerful drug weakening the action of the heart. It is wise to take no medicine, except by the advice of a physician.

Practical Questions

1. Name some narcotics. 2. Tell how tobacco is made. 3. What is the poison in tobacco? 4. How does smoking tobacco harm the young? 5. Why is the smoking of cigarettes especially harmful? 6. Why should tobacco not be chewed? 7. How is opium secured? 8. What is morphine? 9. What is the danger in using drugs? 10. How is the drug habit caused? 11. Why should you not use paregoric or soothing sirup? 12. What is a patent medicine? 13. Why is it wrong to use patent medicines? 14. Can a patent medicine cure consumption? 15. How much is spent yearly for patent medicines?

Suggestions for the Teacher

A very interesting experiment showing the poison in tobacco, may be performed as follows: Secure the stump of a cigar or any small piece of tobacco and boil it five minutes in a little water. Pour this water into a quart or half-gallon jar of water containing a fish, tadpole or any other water-breathing animal and note how soon the creature goes to sleep and then dies.

CHAPTER IX

THE BLOOD AND ITS PASSAGE THROUGH THE BODY

The Need of Blood.—The food, after being digested in the intestine, must be carried to all parts of the body to feed the organs. This is done by the blood constantly flowing in tubes, some of which collect the food from the intestine.

The dead or worn out parts of the body, in the arms, legs and elsewhere, are taken up by the blood and brought to the lungs, kidneys and sweat glands. These organs remove the waste from the blood. The blood is also needed to carry the oxygen of the air from the lungs, to the working cells in all regions of the body.

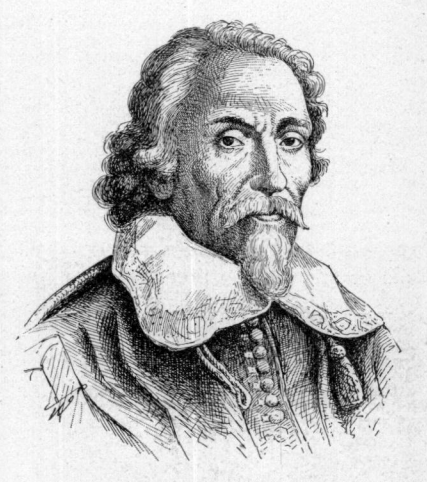

FIG. 48.—William Harvey

The important fact that blood circulates through the body was discovered by William Harvey in 1628.

Parts of the Blood.—The blood is made of tiny cells

THE BLOOD AND ITS PASSAGE THROUGH THE BODY 79

called *corpuscles*, and a liquid named *plasma*. The plasma is almost as clear in appearance as water, but the blood looks red because of the millions of red corpuscles present.

Very soon after blood runs from cut vessels it forms into a jellylike mass. This is called a *clot*. Its formation is known as the clotting of the blood. It is by this means, and the squeezing together of the cut part of the blood tube, that nature stops the flow of blood.

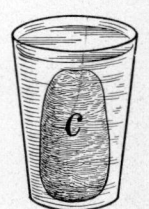

FIG. 49.—This glass was caught full of blood at the slaughtershop, and left standing in a cold room over night. The clot *c*, floats in the serum.

A clot is caused by *fibrin* a threadlike substance which forms in shed blood and entangles the corpuscles. By putting the clot in a cloth and washing and squeezing it in a pan of water, the white fibrin may be washed clear of the corpuscles.

Blood Corpuscles.—These tiny bodies are of two kinds, the red, and the white. The *red corpuscles* have the form of deep saucers or cups, and are five hundred times as numerous as the white ones.

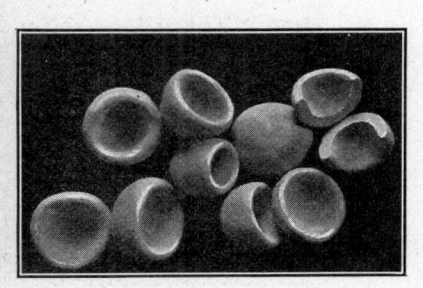

FIG. 50.—Red corpuscles, one of which is cut into halves. Much enlarged.

The *white corpuscles* often like little balls, change their shape almost constantly, and often creep out of the blood tubes and among the tissues. A single drop of blood contains more than a million corpuscles. Many die every hour, and new ones are being formed within the bones and also by small bodies called lymph nodes.

Use of Blood Corpuscles.—The *red corpuscles* are like little boats. They carry oxygen to every cell in the body and carry away much of one kind of waste, known as carbon dioxide. An important part of a red corpuscle is iron. It is shaped like a deep saucer and can carry a larger load than if it were of the form of other cells in the body. Its true form has only lately been discovered. The *white corpuscles* help to clot the blood in a wound. They remove unnecessary tissue, such as the lump formed by the healing of a broken bone. Their greatest duty is to act as soldiers, defending the body from bacteria, which they can destroy in large numbers. A white blood corpuscle has been seen to eat a dozen bacteria in a few minutes. The pus, or white matter, in a sore is largely made of dead white corpuscles, which rushed there to kill the bacteria, but were themselves overcome by the bacteria.

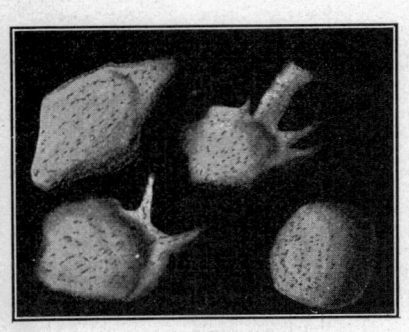

FIG. 51.—White blood corpuscles. The three at the left are creeping about. Drawn from a drop of blood kept warm under the microscope. Much enlarged.

Blood Plasma.—The plasma is a clear fluid. In addition to floating the corpuscles, it contains food for the

THE BLOOD AND ITS PASSAGE THROUGH THE BODY

cells of the body, and some ashes or waste matter given out by the cells. Like the white corpuscles, it passes out through the small, thin-walled tubes so as to bathe every cell in the body and give it food. At the same time it receives and carries away waste products.

Blood plasma is present only in the living body. When blood has been caught in a glass, a clot forms, and on the following day a clear fluid is seen to surround the clot. This is *blood serum*. It differs from plasma in not having in it the agent causing the blood to clot.

How the Blood Passes through the Body.—The blood is contained in a central organ called the *heart*, and branching tubes named *vessels*. One set of vessels named *arteries* carries the blood from the heart to the head, legs and other parts of the body. Another set of

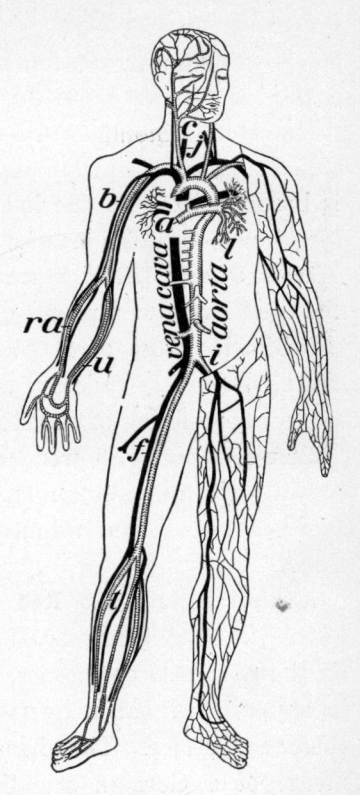

FIG. 52.—Chief veins and arteries of the body. *a*, place of the heart; the veins are in black. On the right side of the picture the veins just under the skin are shown and on the other side the deep vessels near the bones. *b*, vessels to the lungs.

vessels known as *veins* returns the blood to the heart. The veins appear as blue lines beneath the skin on the under side of the wrist.

The small amount of blood oozing out of the tiny tubes called *capillaries* which connect the veins with the arteries, is brought back to the heart by a set of vessels named *lymphatics* or *lymph vessels* (Fig. 56).

How Strong Drink reaches the Blood.—Very little of the food swallowed passes directly from the stomach into the blood. Most of it goes into the intestine. Strong drink, however, quickly enters the transparent blood tubes in the lining of the stomach. Within three minutes after whisky is swallowed some of it may be found in the blood. The greatest amount of alcohol is present in the blood about fifteen minutes after the drink has been taken.

Alcohol Injures the Red Blood Corpuscles.—So far as known, a small quantity of wine or whisky has no effect on the red blood corpuscles. The large amount of alcohol in liquor, often taken by steady drinkers, badly damages these corpuscles. This has been shown by the experiments of a German scientist in 1904. In some cases, when much whisky is used daily, many corpuscles are entirely destroyed, and the person becomes sick because of poor blood.

Alcohol Makes the White Corpuscles Weak.—The germs of disease often get into the body with food and drink, or when the skin is cut and bruised. They are generally prevented from harming the body by the white blood corpuscles, which devour them. Late experiments in

THE BLOOD AND ITS PASSAGE THROUGH THE BODY 83

France have shown that these corpuscles are much weakened when persons use alcoholic drink.

Rabbits into which anthrax germs are put, do not take the disease until they are fed alcohol. Tuberculosis often attacks drinkers when their white blood corpuscles

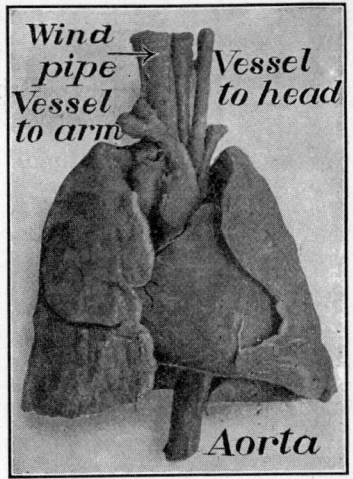

FIG. 53.—The heart between the lungs. From a photograph.

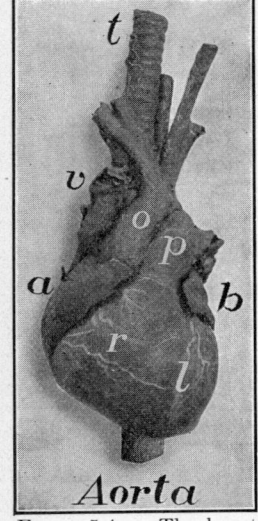

FIG. 54.—The heart from in front. *a,* right auricle; *b,* left auricle; *r,* right ventricle; *l,* left ventricle; *p,* artery to the lungs; *o,* aorta; *v,* vena cava. From a photograph.

have become weakened by the use of alcohol. A noted French scientist has lately said that nearly one half the deaths from tuberculosis are due to alcohol.

The Heart.—The heart is about as large as one's fist, and lies between the lungs in the chest cavity. It has the shape of a strawberry. Its walls are made of muscle, and the cavity within is divided into four parts. The two upper chambers with thin walls are the *auricles.* The two lower chambers with thick walls are the *ventricles.*

The auricles receive the blood from the veins, and pass it to the ventricles, through two openings guarded by valves (Fig. 60). These prevent the blood from flowing backward. Each ventricle by squeezing its walls together forces theblood out into an artery.

The Arteries.—These are the vessels bearing the blood away from the heart. Their walls are made largely of muscle and other elastic tissue. The *lung artery* carries the blood from the right ventricle to the lungs, in which it branches like the limbs of a tree. This branching allows the blood to come in close contact with the air in the richly branching air tubes of the lungs. In this way the blood gets its oxygen from the air.

The main artery through the trunk of the body is the *aorta* receiving the blood from the left ventricle. The aorta gives off more than a score of branches to the head, arms, ribs, digestive organs, and legs. Each of these branches divides again and again like the limbs of a tree, until they become smaller than hairs. At the end of these hairlike branches is a network of still finer tubes, called *capillaries*. These join the arteries with the veins (Fig. 52).

The Veins.—The veins beginning in little branchlets receiving the blood from the capillaries, unite into larger and larger vessels until there are but two chief veins in the trunk of the body. One of these great veins, as large as the thumb, receives the blood from the head and arms and empties it into the right auricle of the heart. The other vessel, lying just in front of the backbone, receives the blood from the legs and digestive organs, and carries it also into the right auricle.

The blood is brought to the left auricle from the lungs by several *lung veins*. This is called *arterial blood*, because it has just received oxygen from the air in the lungs, and cast off its carbon dioxide. All other veins carry *venous blood*, which is rich in carbon dioxide, but contains little oxygen. All arteries, except the lung artery, carry arterial blood, which is rich in oxygen.

The Capillaries.—The capillaries form the network of tiny tubes joining the ends of the arteries with the beginning of the veins. They are so abundant everywhere in the flesh, that a pin cannot enter it without piercing one. Their wall is thinner than the thinnest tissue paper, so that the food in the blood can pass through to feed the cells of the body.

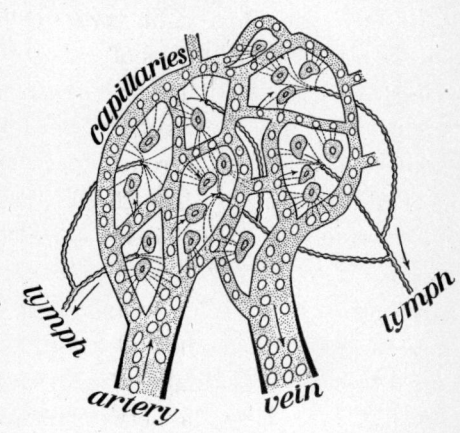

FIG. 55.—Blood plasma passing out of the capillaries to feed the cells. It is there taken up by the lymph vessel.

The oxygen also passes out of the blood through the walls of the capillaries to supply the tissues, and at the same time carbon dioxide and other waste enter the blood.

Some of the blood plasma and white corpuscles pass out of the capillaries and are not able to return to them. They are taken up by another set of tubes called lymph vessels (Fig. 57).

The Lymph Vessels or Lymphatics.—These are numerous small tubes, beginning with mouths opening into the many spaces among the muscles and just under the skin. The tubes unite into larger and larger vessels until there are but two main ones. These lead into the veins in the neck. The largest lymph vessel is the left *thoracic duct*. This is about the size of a lead pencil and lies in front of the backbone.

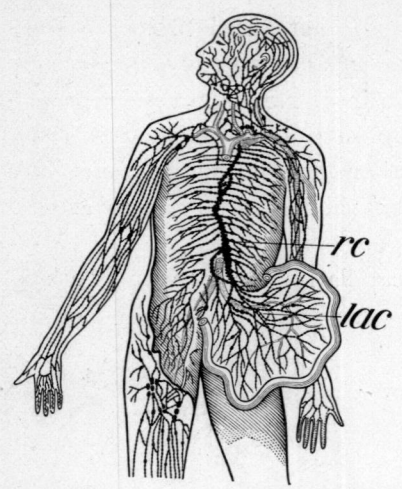

FIG. 56.—The lymph vessels of the body. *rc*, the thoracic duct; *lac*, the lacteals taking the lymph and fatty part of food from the intestines.

That part of the blood escaping from the capillaries together with some waste matter from the cells of the body, forms the lymph conveyed by the lymph vessels.

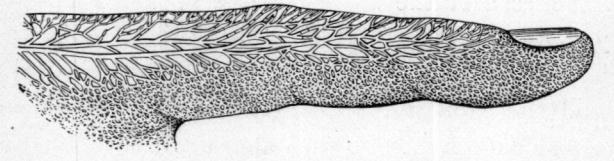

FIG. 57.—Lymph vessels just under the skin of the finger.

Poisons or medicines introduced under the skin are taken up by the lymph vessels. Bacteria in the mouth and digestive canal may enter the soft tissues and then get into the lymph vessels. The lymph vessels pass through bodies named *lymph nodes* or *glands*. These are able to destroy many bacteria.

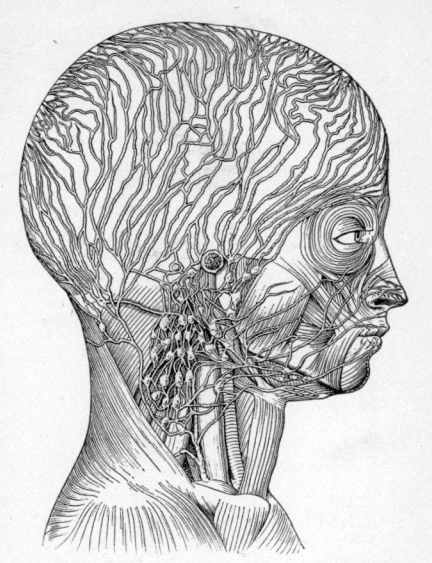

How the Blood Feeds the Body.—The tiny capillaries and lymph vessels in the millions of villi sticking out into the cavity of the small intestine drink in the liquid food. It is then carried by the blood to the liver or by the lymph vessels to the veins in the neck. By the veins of the liver and those of the neck, the food reaches the heart, which sends it with the blood through the arteries to all parts of the body. All arteries lead into capillaries which allow the food to pass out through their walls to nourish the body cells.

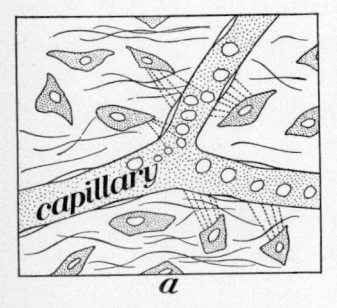

Fig. 58.—Lymph vessels and lymph nodes or glands.

Fig. 59.—Blood plasma passing out of capillary to feed the body cells.

Course of the Blood.—The blood always flows in one direction, because the four valves in the heart close when the blood attempts to go backward. Starting from the left ventricle, the blood goes through the arteries of the body, then passes through the capillaries into the veins of the body, to be returned to the right auricle. From here it flows to the right ventricle to be forced through the arteries to the lungs, from which the veins return it to the left auricle sending it to the left ventricle.

What Makes the Blood Move.—The heart is the main force causing the movement of the blood around within the body. This movement is called the *circulation*. The blood goes from the heart to the toes, and returns in less than one minute. In the arteries it does not flow steadily but in waves. This may be felt by placing the finger lightly on the artery in the wrist at the base of the thumb.

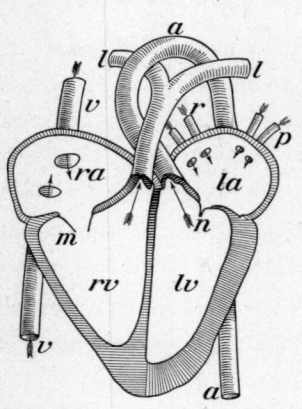

FIG. 60.—Diagram of the heart with its front half removed. *ra*, right auricle; *rv*, right ventricle; *la*, left auricle; *lv*, left ventricle; *a*, aorta; *v*, chief vein of trunk; *r* and *p*, veins from lungs; *l*, arteries to the lungs; *m*, valve open as when blood flows from auricle to ventricle; *n*, valve closed as when blood goes through the aorta.

The beating of an artery is called the *pulse*. It is produced by the squeezing together and the pushing out of the walls of the heart, forming the heart beat. The heart beats in a grown person about seventy times per minute and in babies 140 times each minute.

THE BLOOD AND ITS PASSAGE THROUGH THE BODY 89

The squeezing together of the walls of the ventricles pushes the blood into the arteries because the valves prevent it from flowing back into the auricles. The pushing apart of the walls of the ventricles tends to suck the blood down from the auricles which beat feebly to aid the flow of the blood. The valves at the openings of the arteries from the ventricles prevent the blood from coming back into them. The elasticity of the arteries and the pressure of the muscles on them in moving and breathing, aid in pushing the blood along.

How Exercise Affects the Heart.—After walking up hill, or running for a few minutes, the heart will beat much faster and stronger. This is because more oxygen was needed by the muscles. At every movement of the body oxygen is used up. The hungry tissues cry out for more and order the heart to beat quicker, so that the blood will flow faster, and thus carry more oxygen from the lungs. Very prolonged and violent exercise such as jumping the rope or continuous running, overworks the heart, and may cause sudden death.

Fainting.—In crowded houses where there is much heat and impure air, or because of fright the heart may become weak and beat very slowly. Too little blood is then sent to the head, the person becomes dizzy and falls into a deep sleep. This is called fainting. The person should be laid flat on the back, on the floor, the clothing loosened, and the windows opened wide. A few splashes of cold water in the face are helpful. Recovery usually occurs in a few minutes.

Bleeding from a Wound.—More than a quart of blood

90 THE BLOOD AND ITS PASSAGE THROUGH THE BODY

may be lost without causing death. The flow from an artery is more dangerous than that from a vein, because it runs out with so much more force that a clot cannot form to clog up the break. The flow from an artery is by spurts, while that from a vein is a steady stream.

The flow from a small vein or artery may be stopped by merely tying a clean cloth over the wound. To stop the flow from a larger vessel, a handkerchief or cloth should be tied loosely about the limb and then twisted tight by placing a stick underneath and twisting it around once or twice. If a vein is cut, the cloth should be placed on the side of the wound away from the heart, but if an artery is cut, the cloth must be placed between the wound and the heart.

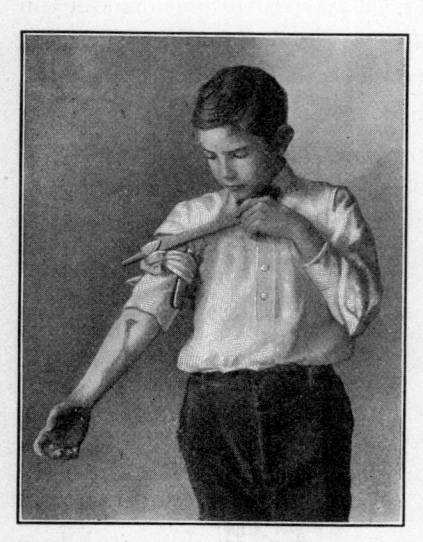

FIG. 61.—Stopping the flow of blood from an artery in forearm. Note that the stick under the handkerchief presses on the main artery near the armpit.

If the wound is made by a dirty nail or instrument, it must be well washed out with water that has been boiled, to kill the bacteria. A few drops of turpentine, alcohol or other germ killer may then be poured on the wound, after which it should be bound up in a clean cloth.

Never put tobacco, cobwebs, or any other dirty material on a cut, or seal it shut with court plaster. Catching cold in a cut means getting bacteria into it. Pus is then often formed and lockjaw or blood poisoning may result.

Exercise and Circulation.—But few people can remain long in good health without exercising one or two hours daily. Persons who take little exercise often feel tired, suffer from headache, and have a poor appetite. This condition is due largely to the sluggishness in the action of various organs, and to the collection of waste matter in the tissues. Medicine gives no lasting help but exercise is a sure cure for this condition.

Exercise makes the heart more active, stimulates greatly the flow of the lymph, so as to carry off the waste matter and hastens the action of many other organs. Swimming, rowing, ball-playing, walking or chopping wood will do more to maintain a healthy blood supply than any medicine.

Alcohol and the Heart.—An unhealthy heart makes a weak body. It has been shown by experiments on animals, as well as by observations on man, that the use of alcohol weakens the heart, causes it to enlarge and changes some of its muscular fibers into fat. It was until lately thought that the heart was stimulated by alcohol, but it is now known that whisky slowly lessens the action of the heart muscle.

It was once customary to give a few swallows of wine or whisky to persons recovering from a fainting or exhausted condition. Lately it has been found that the mere swallowing of anything hot stimulates the heart beat more than the use of alcoholic drinks.

The habitual use of beer causes an overgrowth of heart tissue and an unhealthy formation of fat. In Germany, where much beer is used, hundreds of people die yearly from disease of the heart caused by beer.

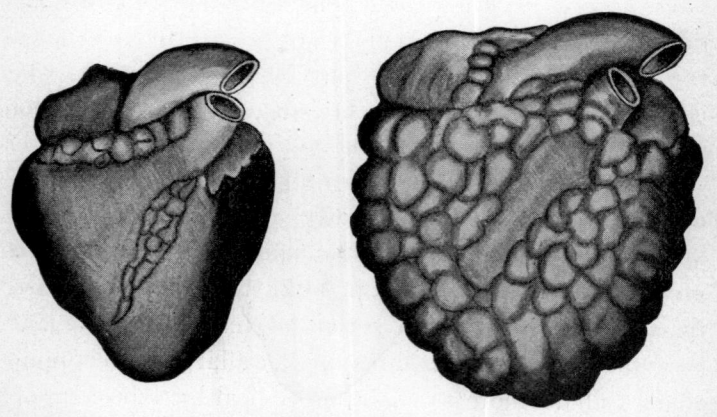

Fig. 62.—Healthy heart on the left and heart of a beer drinker on the right. The irregular white areas are clumps of fat.

Alcohol and the Blood Vessels.—The taking of only one or two tablespoonfuls of whisky will cause the small blood vessels to expand in all parts of the body. Repeated doses of alcohol will keep the blood vessels expanded, and so permit an overcrowding of the blood in many of the organs of the body. This condition is likely to lead to disease of such organs as the liver and kidneys.

The continuous use of alcoholic drinks may also result in a change in the walls of the blood vessels, causing them to become thick and hard. This thickening of the walls later lessens the cavity of the tubes, and so makes the heart work harder to get enough blood through the small channels.

Narcotics and the Blood System.—The use of tobacco by the young often affects the heart so that it beats irregularly. The unsteady tobacco heart is common among boys using cigarettes. A number of candidates for the naval academy are rejected every year, because examination shows that their hearts have been weakened by the use of tobacco, at a time in life when the poison has the greatest effect on the body.

Many persons waste money on the purchase of patent medicines to purify the blood. These medicines frequently contain narcotics, or poisons which harm the blood system, instead of helping it. Blotches and pimples on the skin are not due to disorders of the blood, but to sickness in some organs of the body which need the attention of a trained physician.

Practical Questions

1. Give three uses for the blood. 2. Who discovered the circulation of the blood? 3. Name the two parts of the blood. 4. How is a clot of blood used? 5. Describe the two kinds of blood corpuscles. 6. Of what use are the red corpuscles? 7. Of what use are the white corpuscles? 8. What is blood serum? 9. Name the kinds of blood vessels. 10. How does alcohol injure the blood? 11. Describe the heart. 12. Which cavities receive the blood when it enters the heart? 13. Which vessels carry the blood from the heart? 14. Where does the blood get its oxygen from the air? 15. Name the chief artery in the trunk of the body. 16. Where does the blood enter the veins? 17. How does arterial blood differ

from venous? 18. Of what use are the capillaries? 19. Give the use of the lymph vessels. 20. Explain how the blood feeds the body. 21. Give the course of the blood. 22. What makes the blood flow in the vessels? 23. How many times per minute does your heart beat? 24. What is the remedy for fainting? 25. Explain how the flow from a cut vessel may be stopped. 26. How should a cut be cared for? 27. How does alcohol affect the heart? 28. How does alcohol harm the blood vessels? 29. How does exercise help one to keep well? 30. What effect have cigarettes on the heart?

Suggestions for the Teacher

The teacher who wishes to arouse in the pupils a lasting interest in this wonderful organ of life and have them fully understand how it works, should ask one of the pupils to secure from the butcher shop the entire heart of a calf, pig or sheep. Note the thick-walled artery leading from each ventricle and the several thin-walled veins entering the auricles. By cutting off the lower third of the heart, the cavities of the ventricles and the valves guarding the openings to the auricles may be seen.

CHAPTER X

BREATHING AND ITS USE

What Air is Made of.—Air is a mixture of four parts of nitrogen and one part of oxygen. This may be shown by placing a match head on a bit of floating wood in a pan of water and turning a glass over it as soon as lighted. The burning of the match head will use up all of the oxygen under the glass, and the water will then rise one fifth of the height of the glass to take the place of the oxygen.

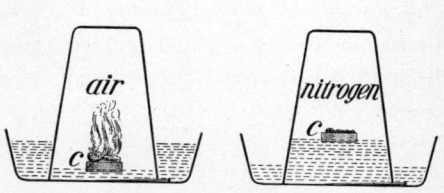

FIG. 63.—Experiment to show amount of oxygen in air. The match heads in burning at the left have used up the oxygen so that the water rises to take its place as shown at the right.

Why We Breathe.
—Air is breathed into the lungs so that the blood can get the oxygen out of it and carry it to the cells of the body. Animals cannot live without oxygen. Even such little creatures as flies must have oxygen supplied to every cell in their bodies. Flies, caterpillars, and all other insects, have tubes branching throughout their bodies to carry air. Openings to these tubes may be seen along each side of the body of a grub or caterpillar. Some animals, such as the fish and crab, which live in water

have gills instead of tubes or lungs to take oxygen into the blood.

The oxygen when within our bodies unites with the food eaten or with the tissues of the body and produces heat and energy. The union of the oxygen with any substance is *oxidation*. The living action of the cells causes oxidation in all parts of the body.

When a match is burned some ashes are left. Slow burning, or oxidation of food and dead flesh in the body leaves some ashes. Much of this is *carbon dioxide*, a heavy gas. This is carried by the blood to the lungs, which breathe it out into the air. We breathe, therefore, to get oxygen into the blood and to cast out carbon dioxide.

The Parts of the Breathing System.—The four chief parts of the breathing or respiratory system are the *nose, throat, windpipe* and *lungs*. The air entering the nose follows the *nasal passages* back to the throat or *pharynx*. Here it enters a tube called the windpipe or *trachea*. This is larger in diameter than the thumb, and three times as long. Its walls are stiffened with gristlelike rings. Its upper part made largely of gristle forms the *larynx* or *voice box*. The windpipe at its lower

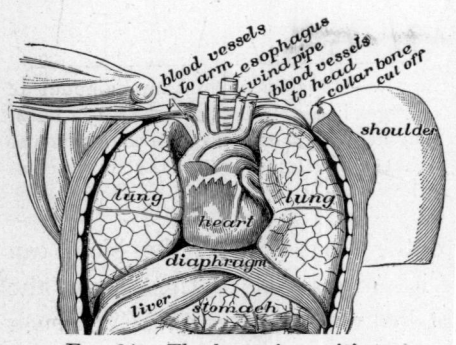

FIG. 64.—The lungs in position.

BREATHING AND ITS USE

end divides into two tubes, the *bronchi,* one of which enters either lung.

The Lungs. — The lungs fill up most of the cavity of the chest. One lies on either side of the heart which is in the middle of the chest. The lungs in animals are called lights because they are spongy sacs and so light as to float when thrown into water. The lungs are really elastic bags consisting of many *tubes* branching to end in the 725,000,000 *air sacs* covered with a fine network of blood capillaries.

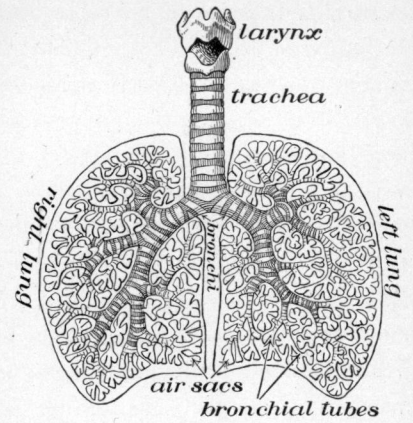

FIG. 65.—Diagram of the air tubes with the lung tissue removed.

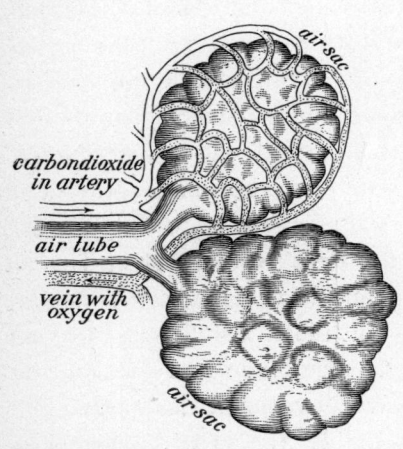

FIG. 66.—Two of the air sacs from the lungs with the network of blood tubes shown about one.

Each tube which branches from the windpipe enters the lung and then divides again and again like the branches of a tree. The small end-branches open into air sacs. The many branching tubes are called *bronchial tubes.*

How we Breathe.—Across the bottom of the chest cavity is a thin muscle named the diaphragm. It arches upward so that its form is like a deep saucer turned upside down. By shortening certain muscles, the diaphragm is stretched so that the center is pulled down. This act, and the pulling up of the ribs forming the sides of the chest, increase the size of the chest cavity and lessen the pressure on the lungs. This causes air to enter the lungs. This act is named *inspiration*. By making the chest smaller the air is forced out of the lungs. This is *expiration*.

Breathing occurs about eighteen times each minute when one is resting, but much oftener during exercise or excitement.

Changes in the Air in the Lungs.—When the air enters the lungs it contains almost no carbon dioxide. When it comes out of the lungs, nearly one twentieth of it is carbon dioxide, and there is one fifth less oxygen than in the entering air. If one breathe a full breath into a wide mouth pint bottle, it will contain so much carbon dioxide that a lighted splinter thrust into it will at once be extinguished. This shows how breathing makes the air of a room impure.

How Oxygen Reaches the Cells of the Body.—The air sacs of the lungs, made of thin transparent membrane, are covered with a network of blood capillaries. Oxygen quickly passes through the membrane and the walls of the capillaries and is received by the little boatlike red corpuscles which float along to the heart. This sends the corpuscles with their load of oxygen out to the capillaries in all regions of the body. The thin walls of the capillaries allow the oxygen to pass out through them to supply the cells.

While the oxygen is passing out of the capillaries to the cells, the carbon dioxide formed in the cells enters the blood through the walls of the capillaries. The blood flows very slowly through the capillaries, so that plenty of time is given for the exchange of these gases. The carbon dioxide, when once in the blood, is carried by the red corpuscles and plasma to the lungs, where it goes out into the air sacs and is then breathed forth from the body. This exchange of oxygen for carbon dioxide in the body is called *respiration*.

How to Make a Drowning Person Breathe.—A person after being under the water two or three minutes stops

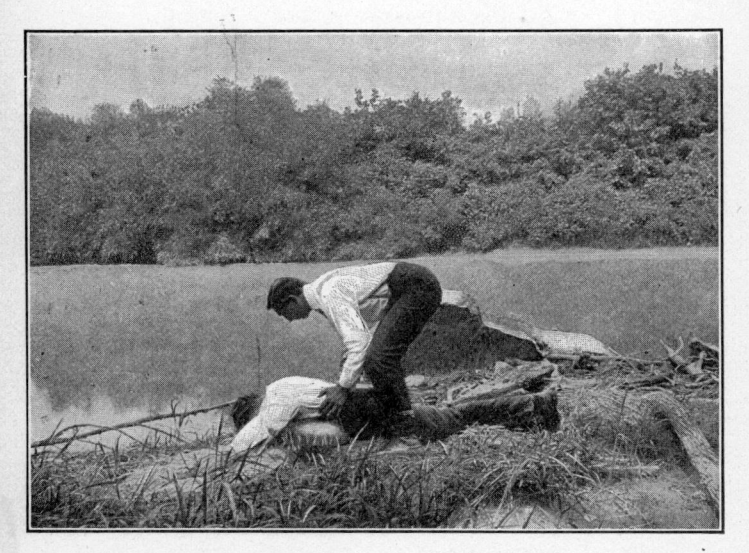

FIG. 67.—The way to make a drowning person breathe.

all efforts to breathe, and appears as if dead. A shock of electricity or exposure to a poisonous gas may also render one unconscious. Such an individual may often be made to breathe again and recover completely by causing artificial respiration in the following manner:

Pull the tongue out between the teeth, as soon as the patient is turned face downward on the ground and place a heavy folded coat or even a piece of sod under the chest. Stand astride him, and with the hands placed on the lower ribs bend forward so as to press in the ribs and force the air out of the lungs. Then straighten your body slowly, keeping the hands on the ribs, while lessening gradually the pressure. This causes the air to enter the lungs. Perform this act about sixteen times per minute. A half hour may be required to restore breathing.

The Voice Box.—The tubelike enlargement at the top of the trachea is the *larynx* or voice box. It is made of several pieces of gristle held together by muscle and other tissue. The largest piece of gristle forms the prominence in the throat, called the *Adam's apple*.

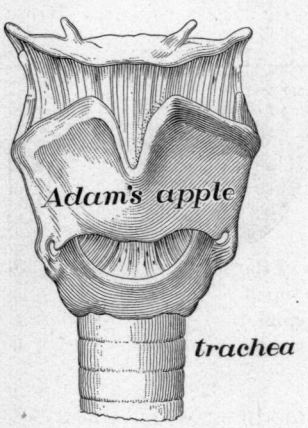

FIG. 68.—The Larynx.

Within the top of the larynx, and stretching from before backward on either side, is a fold of membrane called a *vocal cord*. The narrow opening between the two vocal cords is the *glottis* in front of which stands a small stiffened plate of tissue known as the *epiglottis*. This aids in keeping food out of the windpipe.

The Voice.—Voice is produced either by forcing the breath out, or drawing it in between the stretched vocal cords. The rushing of the air past the vocal cords in the glottis causes them to vibrate like a stretched string when it is struck with the finger. This throws the air into waves in such a way as to make a sound. The higher sounds are produced by tightening the vocal cords by means of muscles pulling on the pieces of cartilage forming the larynx.

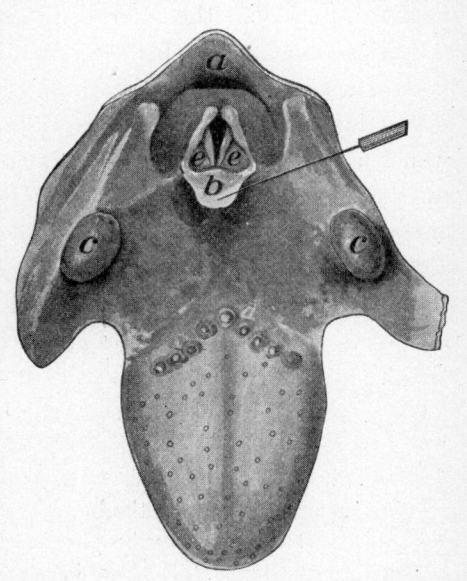

Fig. 69.—View of the upper surface of tongue and into the top of the larynx. *a*, opening to gullet; *b*, epiglottis pulled forward; *e*, is on the outer side of either vocal cord; *c*, tonsils.

The sounds made by the vocal cords are greatly modified into *speech* by the action of the palate, forming the roof of the mouth, and by the tongue, teeth and lips. All animals from frogs to man have vocal cords and would probably be able to talk if they knew how to hold the parts of the mouth and throat in the proper position.

Training the Voice.—The quality of the voice may be much changed by the way in which the teeth, tongue, lips and palate are held. Every boy and girl should try to cultivate a soft, clear voice and avoid the harsh rasping sounds which make one's talk unpleasant. The success of business men is sometimes largely due to their amiable manner and pleasant tone of voice.

The habit of mumbling or speaking indistinctly is one which if not overcome during school days may be a great hindrance to success. In talking the mouth should be opened quite wide, the lips moved firmly and the soft palate stretched so as to produce clear and distinct tones. When one is hoarse, the voice should be used as little as possible. A valuable training for the voice is reading aloud.

Practical Questions

1. Of what does air consist? 2. Why do animals breathe? 3. Of what use is oxygen in the body? 4. Name the parts of the breathing system. 5. Describe the lungs. 6. What causes air to run into the lungs? 7. How does the air breathed into the lungs differ from that breathed out? 8. How does the oxygen reach the cells of the body? 9. How does carbon dioxide get from all parts of the body to the lungs? 10. What is respiration? 11. Tell how to perform artificial respiration. 12. When is artificial respiration of use? 13. Describe the voice box. 14. Describe the vocal cords. 15. How is voice produced? 16. What are used besides the vocal cords in making speech? 17. Why should you learn to speak pleasantly and distinctly? 18. How may the voice be trained? 19. Why is it important you should have a pleasant voice? 20. Can you talk distinctly without moving the lips?

CHAPTER XI

AIR AND HEALTH

Preventing Sickness of the Respiratory System.—About a quarter of a million of people die every year in our country from disease of the lungs and throat. A half million others are sick with some ailment of the respiratory system. Much of this misery is due to breathing air full of dust or other impurities. The dust of the street should be kept down by sprinkling. Floors should be oiled or treated with dust-killing substances before being swept. Dust irritates the tender lining of the air tubes and thus opens the way for disease. A damp cloth should be used in dusting furniture, because the dust and disease germs will stick to it and not fly about.

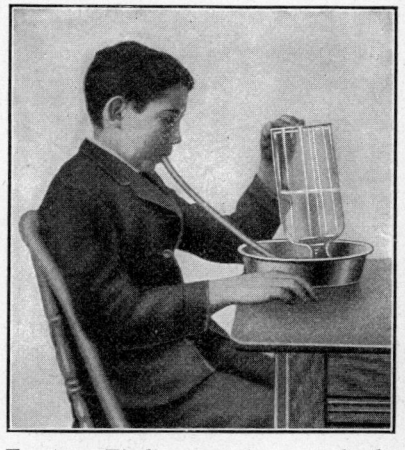

FIG. 70.—Finding out how much the lungs will hold. The bottle full of water was turned upside down with its mouth under water in the pan. The boy blows through the rubber tube extending up into the mouth of the bottle and forces out as much water as possible.

From the inner surface of the nose and all air tubes stick out tiny hairlike projections called cilia. These millions of cilia are always waving up and down in such a way as to move any dust particles outward from the lungs. This keeps the air sacs from being filled up.

Exercising the Lungs.—The lungs of a twelve-year old boy will hold nearly a gallon of air. By effort he can force out at one breath almost three quarts of this. In ordinary breathing, only about one pint comes out at each breath. Many of the air sacs are scarcely used at all and therefore they become weak and liable to disease. The chest instead of being full and round is flat or hollow in front.

Girls and boys should exercise their lungs several minutes each day, by taking in as much air as possible at one breath. They should breathe through the nose so that the air will be warmed and most of the dust caught by the cilia. Swinging the arms back and forth above the head, at the side, behind the back, and in front of the body, strengthens the lungs and wards off disease. In sitting and walking

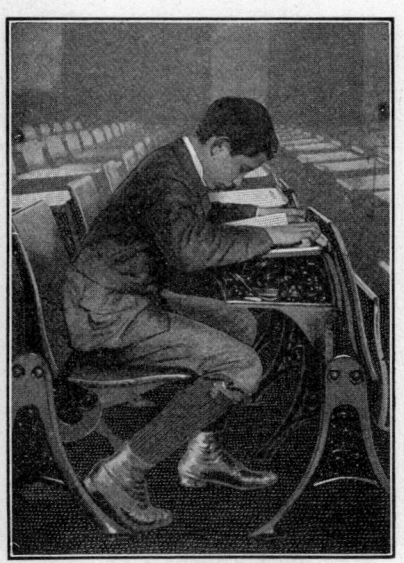

FIG. 71 —How the lungs are squeezed up so that many parts are not used and disease invited.

one should hold the trunk erect and the shoulders thrown back, so that air can reach all parts of the lungs.

Tight Clothing and Breathing.—Bands or other clothing worn tight around the waist or chest do not allow the walls of the chest to expand to their fullest extent. For this reason, the lungs cannot be filled completely with air, and the breathing becomes short and labored. The unused parts of the lungs may become diseased. The clothing about the waist should always be loose, especially in children, and the weight of the garments should be supported by straps over the shoulders.

Need of Supplying Fresh Air in a Room.—Since each person uses a pint of air at every breath, and breathes eighteen times per minute, the air in a room soon becomes foul. It must therefore be exchanged for fresh air. This exchange of foul for fresh air in a room is called *ventilation*. To keep the air of a room pure, twenty cubic feet of fresh air must flow in every minute for each person present.

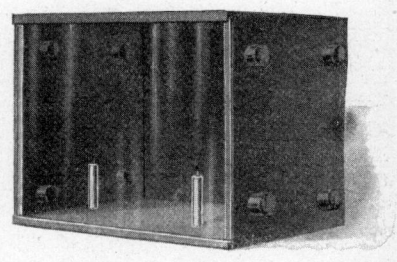

FIG. 72.—A box with two candles and glass front for ventilation experiment. Four corks are in either end for windows. The removal of one cork does not give air enough to permit the candles to burn, but two corks out give sufficient air only when they are at the same end of the box and one above the other.

Impure Air Causes Disease.—About 150,000 persons die of tuberculosis in the United States every year. Many more are sick with the disease. One of the chief causes of this illness is impure air. The air of any room containing one or more persons becomes impure in a few minutes, unless some way is provided for the fresh air to enter.

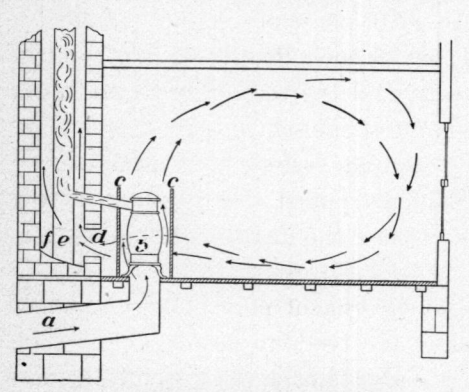

FIG. 73.—Ventilating a rural school. Cold air flows up through the pipe *a*, and is heated by stove *b*, enclosed in sheet iron *c*. The smoke stack *e* warms the air about it in brick flue *f* and thus draws the foul air through the opening *d*.

Some years ago a tribe of Indians in Iowa, who were in good health, were persuaded to leave their tents and dwell in small houses. As a result of the impure air in the poorly ventilated houses, about one half of the Indians now have tuberculosis, and the tribe is rapidly dying off from this disease. Living in impure air weakens nearly all organs and prepares them for disease. Schools that are well ventilated have less than one half as many pupils absent on account of sickness as those with poor ventilation.

Ventilation and Colds.—The air in rooms not well ventilated is usually very dry. This causes the sweat to pass off from the body rapidly and carry with it heat, so that the room seems cold when it is really of a proper temperature.

A room with pure air at sixty-eight degrees will feel warmer than a room with impure dry air at seventy-two degrees. The change from the dry heated air to the moist cool air out doors is a common cause of a cold in the head, often called *catarrh*. In fact the over heated and poorly ventilated room is a frequent cause of all sorts of colds.

How to Ventilate the School Room.—Many children are made tired and sick, and the teacher cross and unfit for duty by the impure air of the schoolroom. All schoolhouses should have a regular system of ventilation but many have not. Windows pulled down from the top give poor ventilation, because the impure air is heavy and near the floor.

The following simple experiment may be tried to show that impure air is heavy and tends to keep near the floor. Breathe two or three times into each of two pint or quart bottles with mouths about an inch in diameter. Then hold one with mouth downward and let the other remain upright. At the end of two minutes, the first one will be free of impure air, so that a lighted stick thrust into it will continue to burn. After ten minutes the upright bottle will contain so much impure air that the lighted stick thrust into it will be at once extinguished.

Animals cannot live and nothing can burn where there is much carbon dioxide.

Several windows raised two or three inches from the bottom and pulled down as much from the top on the same side of the room, give the best ventilation where there is no special provision for ventilating. Drafts must be kept off the children by placing a board slanting inward at the bottom of the window. The fresh air enters at the bottom, sweeps the impure air along to the other side of the room, where it is carried upward and then across beneath the ceiling to the open windows.

A recess of five minutes may be taken every hour when the windows and doors may be opened wide to admit fresh air. Care should be exercised that the room is not made too cold. Children can do nearly twice as much work in a room well ventilated as in one poorly ventilated.

Ventilation in the Home.—The tired, dull, unhappy feeling which often comes on people, especially in the winter season, is frequently the result of impure air. If the home is not heated by hot air brought by pipes from a furnace supplied with a fresh air duct leading from the outer air, a window should be kept open a little at the top and bottom in the living room.

In the sleeping rooms, even in the coldest weather, one window should be open at least a foot, both at the top and bottom. Drafts should not blow on the sleeper. Plenty of covers must be used, and a cap may be worn to keep the head warm. If all people lived in fresh air, there would be but few cases of consumption, and much less sickness from other diseases.

Colds in the Head.—Most children during the winter catch cold in the head. The air passages in the nose become filled up with a white substance called *mucus*. The glands in the mucous membrane lining the nose form this.

These head colds, or catarrh, are usually due to wet feet, sitting in drafts, staying in rooms with dry and impure air, sleeping with the windows closed, or breathing through the mouth instead of the nose. The best remedy is to avoid what caused the evil. A little vaseline put into the nostrils and snuffed up will give some relief. Never use catarrh powders without consulting the family physician. Many of them contain cocaine or other harmful drugs. They may give relief for a short time, but are likely to ruin the health.

Adenoids or Nose Sponges.—Adenoids are spongy growths of the mucous membrane, in the back part of the nose. They are present in very many children. They prevent free nose breathing by clogging the air passages, and may cause partial deafness by shutting up the opening of the tube leading from the throat to the ear.

Abundant adenoid growths sometimes injure the mind by pressing on the blood vessels leading to the brain. Frequent colds in the head, nasal tones, mouth breathing, projecting upper jaw, and inattention are some of the signs that adenoid growths are present. They are easily removed by a physician.

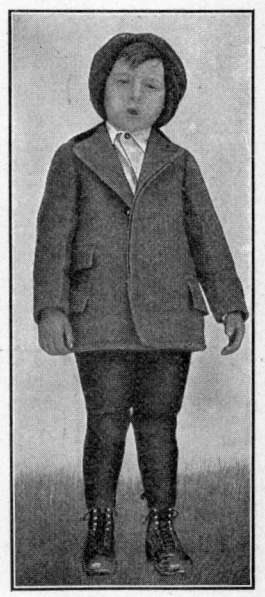

FIG. 74.—Expression of a boy with adenoids. He kept his mouth open day and night.

The *tonsils* which are small useless bodies, one on either side of the tongue, sometimes become much enlarged. They should then be removed as they permit disease germs to enter through them to the blood.

Effect of Alcohol on the Lungs.—The habitual use of alcohol in any form is liable to weaken the lungs so that disease germs can readily get a foothold in them. Pneumonia is not only more likely to attack a drinker than an abstainer, but is more likely to kill him.

Much use of alcoholic drink renders the lungs an especially easy prey to the bacteria of tuberculosis. In many sanatoria for consumptives, there is a large number of patients who have been accustomed to use strong drink. The International Congress at Paris declared that one way to fight tuberculosis is to put down the use of alcohol.

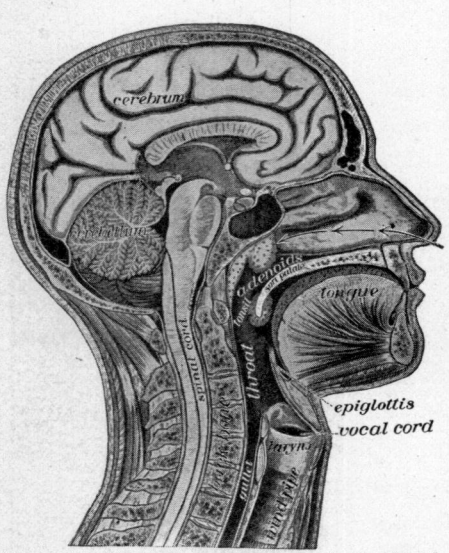

FIG. 75.—Vertical section through the head to show adenoids. Arrows show the course of the air breathed through nose.

Tobacco and the Lungs.—Tobacco has a much less serious effect upon the lungs than alcoholic drink. Habitual users of tobacco, while young, have been known to gain one fourth less in chest girth during four years than those not using the weed. The smallness of the chest would, of course, prevent the full development of the lungs.

In smoking cigarettes, the habit of inhaling the smoke is a bad one, because it allows the nicotine to get into the

AIR AND HEALTH

lungs. Here much more of it can be absorbed than in the throat and mouth, since the thin walled capillaries lie very near the surface on which the poison lodges.

To show how quickly the poison is absorbed into the blood, the following experiment may be performed: The tobacco from three cigarettes is boiled a few minutes in a cup of water to draw out the nicotine. The poisoned water is then poured into a quart of pure water containing a small fish. The narcotic effect of the tobacco causes the fish to go to sleep in about twenty minutes, and about ten minutes later death results. The poison of the tobacco passes into the fish through the gills on either side of the head. They consist of three or four stiff arches bearing fine threads of tissue filled with thin walled blood vessels. The gills are the breathing organs of the fish.

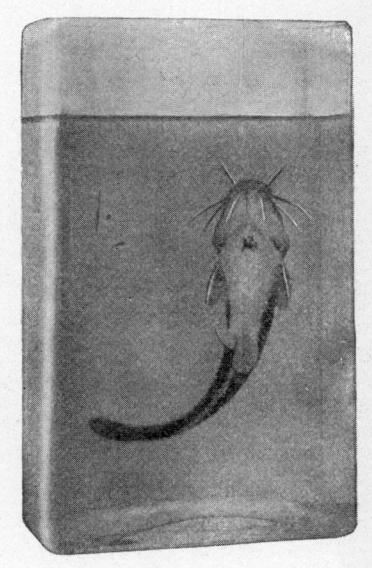

FIG. 76.—This fish died in a half hour from the poison of three cigarettes being placed in its swimming tank.

Practical Questions

1. Why should you try to prevent dust in sweeping? 2. Why are rugs better than nailed-down carpets? 3 How much air do the lungs hold? 4. How much air is taken in by an ordinary

breath? 5. Why should all parts of your lungs be exercised? 6. Why is tight clothing about the chest or waist harmful? 7. What is ventilation? 8. Give facts showing that impure air causes disease. 9. Why is it healthful to have a pan of water on the radiator or stove? 10. Explain how the school room may be ventilated. 11. Why does a lighted candle covered by a quart jar cease burning within a minute? 12. How should a sleeping room be ventilated? 13. What causes cold in the head? 14. What are adenoids? 15. What harm do they cause? 16. How does alcohol affect the lungs? 17. In what way does tobacco hurt the lungs? 18. Describe the experiment showing how tobacco poison hurts a fish. 19. Why is it very injurious to inhale tobacco smoke? 20. Why may much use of tobacco by the young cause tuberculosis later?

Suggestions for the Teacher

The most important lesson a teacher can impress upon the pupils is the need of fresh air to maintain health. Some of the boys can get a valuable exercise in manual training by constructing such a box as is shown in Figure 71. With this box it may be clearly shown that the candles burn strong or weak accordingly as there is much or little fresh air admitted by pulling out the corks. In much the same way the body grows strong or weak according to the amount of fresh air breathed into the deepest parts of the lungs.

CHAPTER XII

CLEANLINESS AND WARMTH

Dead Parts and Waste Matter.—Portions of each cell in the body are constantly wearing out and dying. Whatever is dead must be removed from the system, so that it will not become clogged up.

Considerable matter for food is taken by the blood to all regions of the body, where much of it is oxidized or burned to keep the body warm and furnish energy. The ashes resulting from the burning of this food must be taken away or the body would become filled up like a stove that was never raked or cleaned.

How Ashes and Waste are Removed from the Body.—The ashes remaining from the burning of the food consist largely of carbon dioxide and water. The carbon dioxide is carried by the blood to the lungs, which throw it out in breath. Some of the water is taken

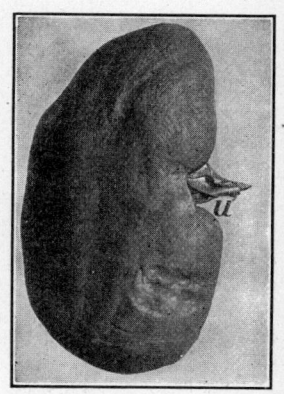

FIG. 77.—One of the kidneys. Half natural size.

from the blood by certain glands in the skin which form the sweat, much water is also removed from the blood by the two kidneys lying back of the stomach. The kidneys

114   CLEANLINESS AND WARMTH

also collect from the blood and discharge from the body the waste flesh. This comes from the worn-out and dead parts of any organ, and would poison the body if it were not carried away daily.

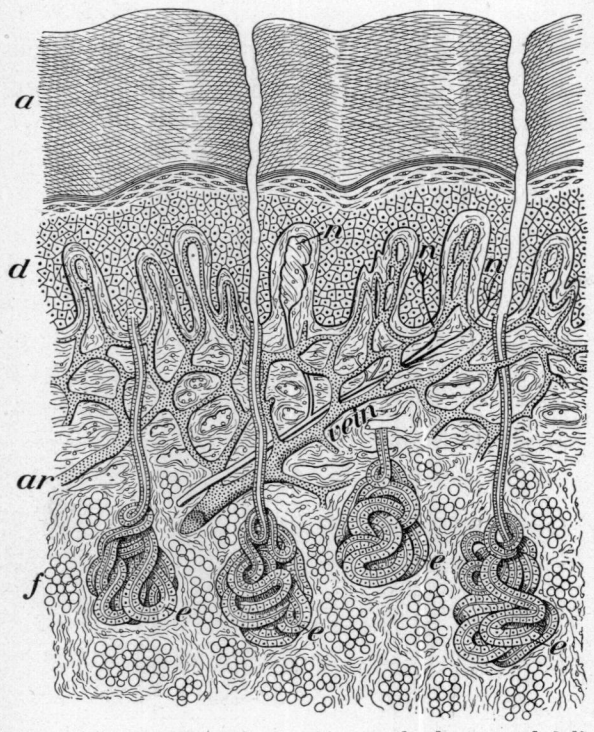

Fig. 78.—A thin slice through the skin. *a*, dead part and *d*, live part of the epidermis; *ar*, artery; *e*, sweat glands; *n*, nerve endings. Much enlarged.

The liver also removes some waste from the blood and discharges it as part of the useful bile into the intestine. The four chief organs, therefore, concerned in keeping the body clean within, are the lungs, liver, kidneys and skin.

The Skin.—The skin is an elastic covering stretched over the muscles and fatty tissues. It is bound loosely to these by a threadlike network called connective tissue. The chief use of the skin is to support the sense organs of feeling, to regulate the temperature of the body and to protect the delicate parts lying beneath.

The skin is made of two layers, each of which has a different use. The layer on the surface is known as the *epidermis* or *scarf skin*, while the deep layer is called the *dermis* or *true skin*.

The Scarf Skin or Epidermis.—This portion of the skin contains no blood vessels, but in the deeper part are nerve endings for feeling. It is made of several layers of cells. The top ones are nearly flat, dry, dead and scaly, and are being constantly rubbed off. A frog or snake sheds the upper layer of its scarf skin in one piece three or four times a year.

The chief use of the scarf skin is to protect the underlying tender tissues and keep bacteria from entering the blood. In regions of the body where the skin is much in contact with hard objects, as on the palms of the hands and the soles of the feet, the scarf skin becomes very thick and hard.

Corns.—Much pressure or friction on any part of the foot by a shoe is likely to produce a corn. This is a thickening of the epidermis in one spot, so that it presses on the tender true skin.

One should never wear tight shoes, or those with narrow

toes not allowing the foot to keep its natural shape. A corn once formed is difficult to remove. The use of a corn ring such as may be purchased from the druggist, to prevent entirely the pressure of the shoe on the tender spot, is a great relief. The occasional shaving off of the top of the corn with a clean knife after the foot has been soaked a few minutes in hot water, is a helpful remedy.

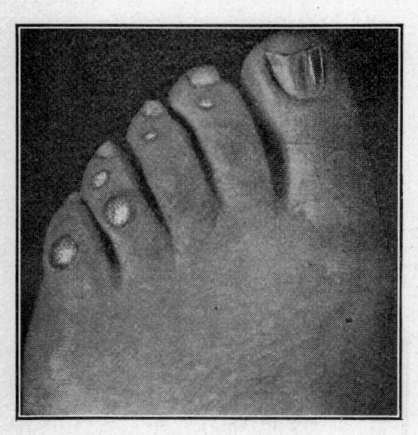

FIG. 79.—Corns on the two outer toes resulting from tight shoes.

Blisters and Warts.—Blisters are caused by any irritation such as continued rubbing or pinching. They are formed by a pushing out of the upper layer of the epidermis with a collection of lymph which oozed from the blood capillaries. Removing the cause will permit a cure to take place in a few days.

Warts are overgrowths of the epidermis including an upgrowth of the true skin. Their cause is unknown. They are not produced by touching toads. Fortune tellers cannot remove them by saying words. They are easily removed by a physician.

Tanning and Freckles.—Every one has some color in the skin. The red color is due to the blood in the vessels of the true skin, showing through the thin scarf skin. Any exercise or emotion causing the gorging of these vessels in the cheeks, produces blushing.

The brown hue of the skin results from a dark coloring matter known as *pigment*. This is present in many organs of the body. The pigment is conveyed into the deepest part of the scarf skin by the white blood corpuscles. Exposure to the sun causes these corpuscles to transfer an abundance of the pigment from the deeper tissues to the skin. When the corpuscles deposit the pigment in patches, freckles are formed. Some races, such as the African, have much more pigment in the skin than others. Sun baths are healthful.

The True Skin.—This is thicker than the scarf skin and is of far more importance. It is richly supplied with nerves and blood vessels, and contains the sense organs of feeling, and the sweat glands. By means of all these structures, the true skin is able to help much in regulating the temperature of the body.

How the Body Heat is Regulated.—The temperature of the body is about ninety-eight degrees. It remains the same summer and winter when one is in health. The body will be just as warm in an ice house as in a hot room. This is due to the heat regulating machinery.

In the presence of cold, the vessels of the skin lessen in size so that less blood can come to the surface to be cooled and to furnish sweat. The cold feeling on the skin is carried by nerves to the inner part of the body which sends orders by other nerves to make the muscles in the walls of the blood tubes squeeze up tighter. In warm weather, the vessels of the skin enlarge and receive much blood so that it may be cooled by the air touching the skin. At the same time this extra supply of blood at the surface enables the sweat glands to throw out a large amount of sweat. The drying up of this sweat cools the body, because the heat passes off into the air with the sweat.

The Sweat Glands.—Each of the 2,500,000 sweat glands consists of a tube whose lower end is rolled up into a ball. The openings of the tubes on the surface of the body are the *pores*. These appear under a common magnifying glass as little pits on the ridges in the palms of the hands. The real gland is deep in the true skin and is surrounded by capillaries from which it gets the salty water and small amount of solid matter to make the sweat.

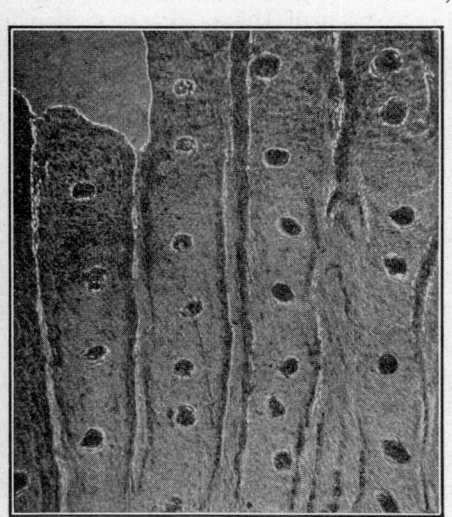

Fig. 80.—Photograph of a tiny bit of the palm of the hand, showing the openings of the sweat glands.

The sweat glands are scattered throughout the skin of the entire body. Hard work on a very warm day may make them give out three quarts of sweat, but the average amount of sweat brought forth daily is only one pint. The sweat often called *perspiration* contains a little waste matter but its chief use is to cool the body.

Keeping the Skin Clean.—Many people wash their hands and face several times daily, because they are soiled by dust and dirt easily seen. Much of the waste matter thrown out by the glands over the entire surface of the skin cannot be seen, but unless it is washed off at least once or twice a week, the person is likely to have an unpleasant odor. As some parts of the body, such as the feet, have much excretion given out by the glands, they should be washed daily.

The hands should always be thoroughly washed by using soap and hot water, just before eating or handling food to avoid germs of disease. The habit of cleanliness is one of the many good habits which everyone should form while young. If the hands become chafed or rough, a little glycerine or cold cream rubbed on them once or twice daily after washing will be helpful.

Bathing.—Bathing is useful not only for the sake of cleanliness, but for making the body strong and healthy. A cold bath taken as soon as one is out of bed in the morning is very helpful to most people, in preventing colds and increasing the appetite. It wakes up the nervous system, makes the heart work faster, and the lungs take in fuller breaths. The room should be warm and the water should have a temperature of sixty or seventy degrees. The cold plunge or shower bath should not last longer than one minute.

If no tub or shower is convenient for use, two or three minutes may be spent in applying cold water to the body with a sponge or towel while standing in a pan or bowl to receive the drippings. As soon as the cold bath is finished, the body should be well rubbed with a coarse towel.

120 CLEANLINESS AND WARMTH

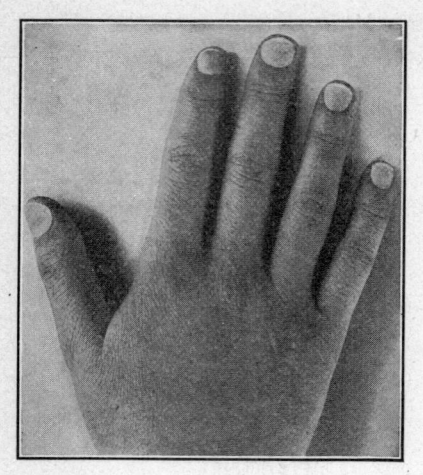

Fig. 81.—Hand with nails properly cared for.

The Hot Bath.—Babies, invalids and some others who cannot use a cold bath, may have a hot bath. This is also stimulating but does not prevent colds. One should not go into the cold out door air, in less than an hour after a hot bath, as a cold may result. It is generally best, therefore, to take the hot bath at bed time.

The Complexion.—The color of the skin may vary much, but in health it should be smooth and soft. If pimples and blackheads occur, it is because some organs of the body are not doing their work properly. A breaking out on the skin of babies and also older persons is often due to improper care of the digestive organs. The condition may some-

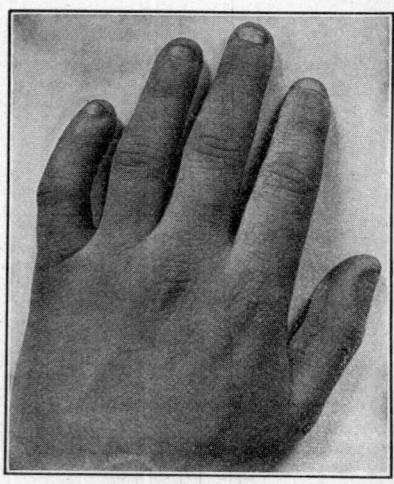

Fig. 82.—Hand of boy who chewed off the ends of his nails causing stubby fingers.

times be helped by eating less meat and sweets, by chewing the food more thoroughly, and by taking plenty of exercise and fresh air.

The Nails.—The nails are made from a hardened part of the epidermis. When properly cared for they add much to the usefulness and appearance of the hand. Biting the ends of the nails off makes blunt and unshapely fingers. The ends of the nails should be filed off daily or cut weekly. The dirt should be removed from beneath them each time after washing the hands, and not when it is in a dry state.

The Hair.—The base of each hair is held in a little sac formed by the dipping down of the epidermis. At its bottom is a tiny knob from which a new hair grows when the old one is pulled out or drops away. By the side of the hair sac are one or two oil glands, giving out an oily fluid into the sac near its top. This keeps the hair soft. No other hair oil should ever be used.

To avoid dandruff, the scalp should be thoroughly washed with soap and warm water once or twice a month. The hair should be dried before going out of doors in the cold. The hair should be combed daily, or whenever it becomes untidy, and little or no water used on it.

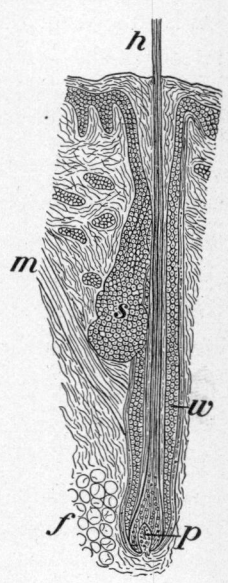

FIG. 83.—A section through the root of a hair. *s*, oil gland; *w*, hair sac; *p*, knob from which the hair grows.

Gray Hair and Baldness.—After middle life the coloring matter often leaves the hair, and it then becomes gray, because the hollow center is filled with air. There is no way of preventing this. Hair dyes should not be used. Some of them contain poison.

Baldness often occurs after the age of forty. None of the much advertised preparations will prevent baldness. Daily massaging or pinching and rolling of the scalp between the fingers for a few minutes will keep the glands and blood vessels active, and thus prevent baldness in some cases.

Bruises and Cuts.—A bruise is a swelled and bluish-colored spot on the skin caused by a blow from something not sharp. The swelling is due to the lymph or watery part of the blood which has oozed through the walls of the hurt blood tubes. The best remedy is to apply a cloth wrung out of very hot or very cold water. It should be changed every three or four minutes for a half hour or more.

A cut is a break in the skin. Even a slight cut, especially if the flesh is torn, may result in a serious sickness, such as lockjaw or blood poisoning. A wound is made sore and white matter called pus produced by bacteria. Every cut or break in the skin should, therefore, be carefully washed with water and cloths which have been boiled to kill the germs. Some germ killer, such as turpentine, alcohol or weak carbolic acid, may then be poured into the cut, after which it should be protected by several thicknessess of a clean cloth.

It was Lord Lister, an Englishman, who discovered in

1870 the method of preventing wounds from getting sore and resulting in blood poisoning. Before his discovery it was common for injured persons to lie in the hospitals day after day while they were slowly being eaten up, or poisoned by germs. By the use of germ killers to cleanse the wounds and clean cotton to keep out the germs, ten times as many seriously wounded persons are saved from death as before the discovery of Lister.

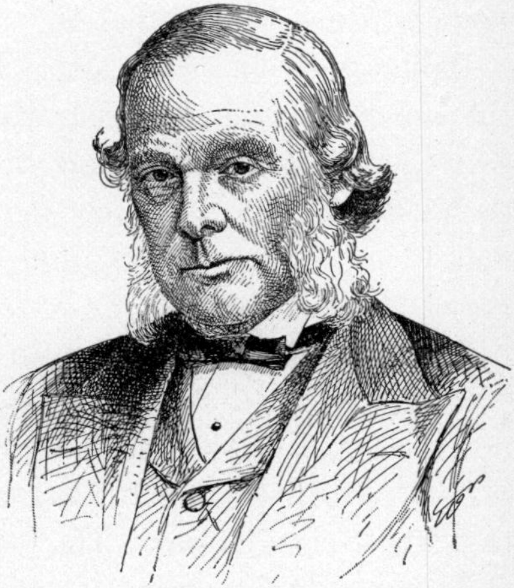

Burns and Scalds.—A good remedy for burns and scalds is *carron oil*. This is made by shaking together in a quart jar a half pint of lime water and the same amount of linseed oil. A clean cloth, folded several times and soaked with carron oil, should be bound at once upon the injured place. Cloths spread with vaseline, or wet with kerosene and applied to the burn, give great relief. Baking soda, moistened to form a paste, and spread on the injured part also relieves the pain.

FIG. 84.—Lord Lister whose discoveries showing how to keep bacteria out of wounds, saves thousands of lives yearly.

Alcohol and the Kidneys.—It has already been shown that the kidneys are important organs in removing from the body what would clog its parts and poison the entire system. It is important therefore, that they should always be in a healthy condition.

The habitual use of beer, whisky, or wine generally produces a change for the worse in the working power of the kidneys. This change comes on so gradually in those accustomed to the use of alcoholic drinks, that the organs are often seriously sick before the victim feels much ill.

Long continued use of alcohol, even that in such weak drinks as beer, often causes part of the kidney tissue to be changed to a fatty substance, and part to become hardened. The whole kidney may shrink. It is no longer able to do its work properly and so fails to remove certain wastes from the blood. This may result in rheumatism, or a more serious ailment, known as Bright's disease.

The cells of the kidney, even in those who use strong drink only moderately, sometimes become sick and let part of the albumin, which is a body food in the blood, escape with the waste matter. This condition is often present for a year or more before the drinker is aware of it. He feels weak, dislikes work, and finally becomes ill enough to consult a physician when it is too late to save his life.

How Alcohol Prevents Keeping the Body Warm.—It has been pointed out that one of the chief uses of the skin is to regulate the temperature of the body. This is done by changing the size of the blood vessels. The size is governed by the nerves causing the loosening of the circular muscles in the walls of the blood tubes. Alcoholic drink even in small quantity acts on the nerves in such a way as to make the blood vessels of the skin enlarge. This allows much blood to come to the surface of the body where it is quickly cooled.

After a drink of liquor in cold weather, the body feels warmer, because a large amount of blood is sent to the skin where the sense organs of heat are located. In reality the body becomes colder as a thermometer will show. This is why drinkers freeze to death more quickly than abstainers.

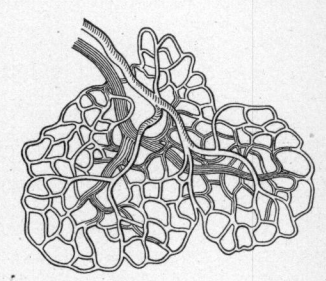

Experience of Sir John Ross with Narcotics.—Ross, in an account of his trip to the Arctic regions, says: "I was twenty years older than any of the officers or the crew, yet I could stand the cold better than any of them, who all made use of tobacco and spirits. I entirely abstained from them. The most irresistible proof of the value of abstinence was when we abandoned our ship, and were obliged to leave behind us all our wine and spirits. It was remarkable to observe how much stronger and more able the men were to do their work when they had nothing but water to drink."

FIG. 85.—The blood vessels of the skin, which alcohol enlarges.

Alcohol and the Skin.—In some persons quite small doses of alcohol taken daily are sufficient to cause changes in the skin. The blood channels are widened, the circulation becomes slower, the working of the glands is interfered with, and eruptions or pimples may appear.

The prolonged and steady use of alcoholic drink causes the blood vessels of the skin to remain permanently enlarged, and thus produce a redness. The flushed face of a drinker in cold weather may take on a dull leaden hue, or a purple bloated look, due to the widened and gorged blood vessels. A roughness of the skin sometimes occurs as a result of failure to throw off the dead epidermis.

Practical Questions

1. What would be the result if dead matter were not removed from the body? 2. Of what does the ashes of burnt food chiefly consist? 3. What do the kidneys remove? 4. What are the four chief organs removing waste from the body? 5. Of what use is the skin? 6. Give the two parts of the skin. 7. Describe the scarf skin. 8. How are corns produced? 9. What is a blister? 10. What causes freckles and tanning? 11. Describe the true skin. 12. What is the temperature of a healthy body? 13. How is the body temperature kept constant? 14. Describe a sweat gland. 15. Of what use is sweat? 16. What care should be taken in keeping the skin clean? 17. Why should a cold bath be taken every morning? 18. What may cause a rough or pimply face? 19. Describe what care should be given the nails. 20. How is a hair fastened in the skin? 21. What will help stop the falling out of the hair? 22. Give the treatment for a bruise. 23. What care should be given a cut? 24. Describe the remedy for burns and scalds. 25. How does alcohol affect the kidneys? 26. How does alcohol affect the skin?

Suggestions for the Teacher

During the study of this chapter the teacher should impress upon the pupils the importance of keeping themselves neat and clean. It is often necessary to give special directions in regard to caring for the hair, hands and nails. The numerous cases of sickness due to touching food with unclean hands, shows the need of washing before eating or handling food.

CHAPTER XIII

CLOTHING AND COLDS

Need of Clothing.—The clothing protects the body from the burning rays of the sun in summer and from cold in winter. It also serves as an ornament. Most people wear too heavy clothing during both summer and winter. In summer too much clothing makes one uncomfortable, and in the winter it may cause colds. It is almost as important to wear the right kind of clothing as to eat the proper kind of food.

Kinds of Clothing.—The four chief kinds of material out of which clothing is manufactured are linen, cotton, wool and silk. The flax plant supplies the threads required for the linen manufactured into shirts, collars and cuffs. The cotton plant furnishes the fibers used in making calico, muslin and other cotton goods. Wool sheared from sheep is woven into woolen cloth for wraps, overcoats and cloth suits. The silk worm changes mulberry leaves into fine silk thread used in making ribbons, neckties and silk dresses.

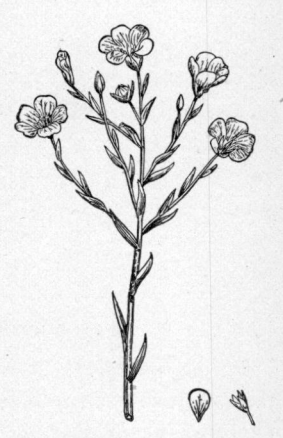

FIG. 86.—The flax plant.

Clothing and Sweat.—Sweat is constantly oozing out on the surface of the body and is absorbed by the clothing next to the skin. The under clothing, therefore, soon becomes soiled and needs to be washed at least once or twice weekly. At night it should be hung up in the room so that the air can dry and purify it.

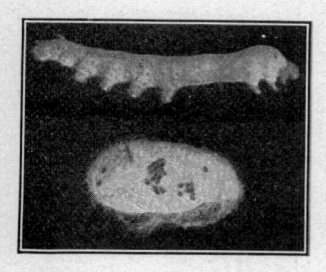

Fig. 87.—The silk worm and its cocoon 50,000 of which are required to make a silk dress.

Sweat is *formed to cool* the body, but it cannot do this unless it soaks through the clothing to the air, so as to carry off the heat. On this account cotton underclothing should be worn in summer. Cotton absorbs sweat much faster than wool and passes it outward toward the air. A newspaper or a rubber coat forms a very warm covering because they do not permit the sweat to be evaporated or the heat to pass outward from the body.

Clothing for Warmth.—Woolen cloth is much warmer than cotton or linen, because it is more loosely woven and thus contains air. This prevents the heat from passing off from the body. Woolen underclothing is therefore better for very cold weather, especially for the old and those who exercise but little.

Lately loose-meshed cotton undergarments have been manufactured in such a way as to hold much air and also absorb the sweat. Such clothing may be worn by well persons both summer and winter. They should, however, protect the body from severe cold by outer wraps.

How Clothing Causes Cold.—Outer wraps and overcoats should always be removed by persons entering a warm room. If they are not laid off, the body becomes covered with sweat which begins to pass off rapidly as soon as one is out in the wind. The body then feels cold and is likely to become chilled. For the same reason heavy clothing should be taken off when one is exercising.

Some persons wear no overcoat during very cold weather, except when riding. This may usually be done with safety if one accustoms his body gradually to the cold, but to leave off the accustomed outer wrap when exposed to severe cold is likely to make one sick. The change from heavy clothing in winter to light weight garments or low-necked dresses often worn at parties, is a common cause of colds, bronchitis and pneumonia. Except in severe cold weather the throat, however, should not be bundled up in furs or muffler, as it may lead to catarrh.

Other Causes of Colds.—The over heated room is a common cause of colds. The temperature of a room should range from sixty-four to sixty-eight degrees. The heat of the room causes the clothing to become moist with sweat, which when one goes out in the wind, quickly evaporates and chills the body. The activity of certain parts of the body concerned in warding off colds is also weakened so the system is overcome by the least chilling.

Many children catch severe colds by exercising until they are warm and then sitting down to cool off. Except in the very warmest weather, one should always put on an extra wrap immediately after exercising and not wait until he feels cool.

Serious colds are frequently contracted by sitting in damp clothing. Moisture conducts the heat away from the body quickly. When the clothes are wet, one must keep exercising or put on heavy wraps to keep warm until dry garments can be secured.

The Catching of Colds.—Smallpox, diphtheria and scarlet fever are known as catching or contagious diseases. Late discoveries show that even a cold may be contagious.

Nansen and his men were in the arctic regions for more than three years, and were exposed to severe cold weather. On some occasions after getting into their sleeping bags, they had to thaw out their frozen clothing by the heat of their own bodies, before they could go to sleep; and yet not one of the number suffered from a cold until they arrived in Norway. Here civilization permitted certain bacteria to reach them and caused an epidemic of colds.

How to Stop Colds.—It is often possible to know when one is beginning to take cold. There is a chilly feeling, a slight heaviness in the head, a roughness in the throat or a watery discharge from the nose. The cold may sometimes be stopped in this stage by taking a hot bath before going to bed and drinking some hot, weak tea or lemonade. One should keep very warm, stay indoors and rest. The food should consist of hot milk, broth, soft boiled eggs and fruit.

Caring for a Cold.—After a cold has been in progress two or three days there is no way of curing it at once. By care, however, the period of its duration may be very much shortened. One should be very warmly clad and if possible avoid going out in the wind. If necessary to leave the house in cold weather, the ears and throat must be covered and the entire surface of the body kept warm to keep too much blood from the inner parts.

The sleeping room should not be very cold, but should be well ventilated. Both the feet and head must be kept warm. A cold cannot be cured by medicines but if the system is out of order, a medicine may help to right it and thus aid the body in curing the cold. Never use the much advertised cough medicines. Many contain chloroform or poisons that will harm the body.

Keeping the Feet Dry.—One of the common causes of sickness is wet feet. No one should sit still with wet feet. Keep exercising until dry stockings and shoes can be secured. Rainproof shoes or rubber overshoes are necessary during the wet season. Shoes to be made rain proof must be oiled weekly. Overshoes should always be removed upon entering a room as they do not permit the sweat to escape.

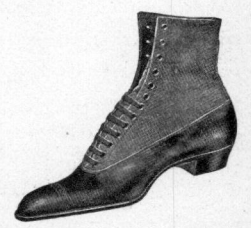

FIG. 88.—A sensible shoe, which does not squeeze the foot.

Relation of Clothing to Alcohol.— In the bleak winter days the laborer and especially the driver feel cold unless clad from head to foot in proper clothes. These men take a drink of whisky because it makes them feel warm. It really makes their body become colder, because alcohol makes the tiny vessels in the skin enlarge. This act lets more

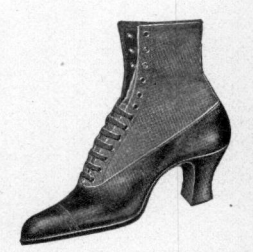

FIG. 89.—An uncomfortable shoe, giving an awkward gait and producing corns.

blood come to the surface, where the cold air quickly cools it. The whole body becomes chilled and severe sickness may result. It is therefore dangerous to make whisky take the place of warm clothing.

Practical Questions

1. Name several kinds of clothing. 2. Why should clothing worn next to the skin be washed frequently? 3. Why should cotton underclothing be worn in summer? 4. Why is woolen clothing warmer than cotton? 5. How may a cold be caused by clothing? 6. How are colds often caught? 7. How may colds sometimes be stopped? 8. Why should the skin be kept warm to prevent a cold from becoming worse? 9. How may a cold sometimes be stopped? 10. Explain how a cold should be cared for. 11. Why cannot alcohol take the place of clothing? 12. Why should you not use the advertised cough medicines? 13. Why is it dangerous to sit with wet feet? 14. Why should high-heeled shoes not be worn? 15. When should overshoes be worn?

The fact that damp garments are likely to be the cause of sickness by taking the heat rapidly away from the body may be shown in the following manner: Fill two warm bottles of the same size with hot water. Wrap one in a dry handkerchief and the other in a wet handkerchief. After a half hour, test with the finger and note the one in the wet cloth is cold while the other is still warm.

CHAPTER XIV

THE BONES

The Use of the Bones.—The bones of the body are used for its support, and also to help it move. The muscles which are made to act by the nerves, pull on the bones so as to move them in any direction one may wish. The bones shield from outward injury the important organs such as the brain, spinal cord, lungs and heart. All of the red blood corpuscles, and many of the white ones, are made in the red bone marrow which fills the many small spaces in the inside of the bones.

Arrangement of the Bones.—There are over two hundred bones in the body. These, joined together in their natural relations, form the bony framework called the *skeleton*. The parts of the skeleton are the *skull*, or bones of the head, the *trunk*, and the *extremities*.

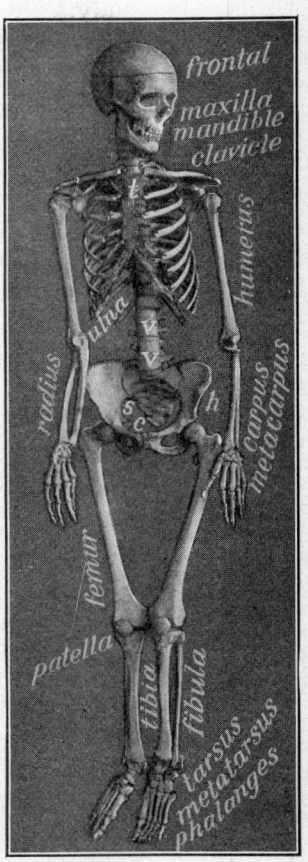

FIG. 90.—The skeleton. *t*, breastbone; *v*, vertebrae; *h*, hip bone. From a photograph.

As the bones in the skeleton of a dog or cat have about the same form and relations as those of man, the bones of these animals often found in the woods or fields may be used for study.

Bones of the Head.—The skull, formed by the bones of the head, is at birth quite incomplete on the sides and top. In these places there are spaces where only membrane separates the brain from the skin. These spaces are not entirely closed with bone until the end of the second year. It is possible, therefore, to cause the death of a baby by a slight stroke on the head.

The Bones of the Skeleton

The Skull or Bones of the Head	Cranium	sphenoid **1**
		frontal **1**
		parietal **2**
		temporal **2**
		occipital **1**
		ethmoid **1**
	Face	nasal **2**
		inferior turbinated **2**
		lachrymal **2**
		maxilla or upper jaw **2**
		mandible or lower jaw **1**
		palate **2**
		malar or cheek bone **2**
		vomer **1**
		hyoid **1**
Bones of the Trunk	Spinal column or backbone	vertebra **24**
		sacrum **1**
		coccyx **1**
	Other bones of the trunk	sternum or breast bone **1**
		ribs **24**
		innominate or hip bone **2**

Bones of the Upper Extremity	Shoulder girdle	clavicle or collar bone 2
		scapula or shoulder blade 2
	Arm	humerus 2
	Forearm	radius 2
		ulna 2
	Wrist	carpal 16
	Hand	metacarpal 10
	Fingers	phalanges 28
Bones of the Lower Extremity	Leg	femur or thigh bone 2
		tibia or shin bone 2
		fibula 2
		patella or knee pan 2
	Ankle	tarsal 14
	Foot	metatarsal 10
	Toes	phalanges 28

There are twenty-two bones in the skull, in addition to the six tiny bones of the ears. The eight bones surrounding the brain form the *cranium*, while the other fourteen make up the *face*. The bony brain case is a quarter-inch thick.

The Bones of the Trunk.—The trunk is made of the *spinal column*, the *ribs*, the *breastbone* and the *hip bones*. These are so arranged as to protect well the internal organs. The spinal column or backbone is made of a chain of twenty-six bones. A canal extends from the top to the bottom of the backbone. This is nearly filled by the spinal cord.

There are twelve pairs of *ribs*. Seven pairs called the *true ribs* are joined to the backbone, and also to the breastbone in front. The five lower pairs of ribs are known as *false ribs* because they are not joined direct to the breastbone.

136 THE BONES

The two outward flaring hip bones with the sacrum between them form a basin called the *pelvis*.

Bones of the Extremities.—The bones of the upper extremity are of similar shape and arrangement to those of the lower extremity, with the exception of the flat shoulder blade or scapula on the back, and the collar bone or clavicle in front of the shoulder. A single bone, the *humerus* reaching from the shoulder to the elbow, forms the *arm*, while two bones, the *ulna* and *radius*, reaching from the elbow to the wrist, make up the *forearm*. The *femur* or *thigh bone* extends from the hip to the knee, and a strong bone, the *tibia* or shin bone, with a slender bone, the

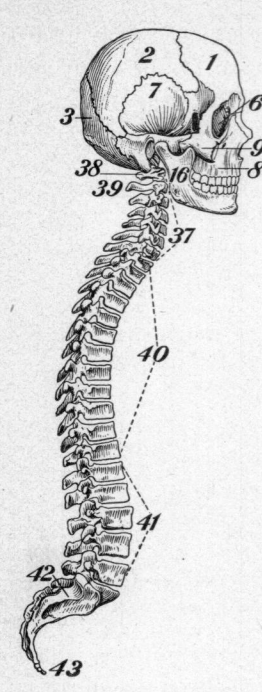

FIG. 91.—Side view of skull and spinal column 1, frontal; 2, parietal; 7, temporal. Note the separate bones of the backbone

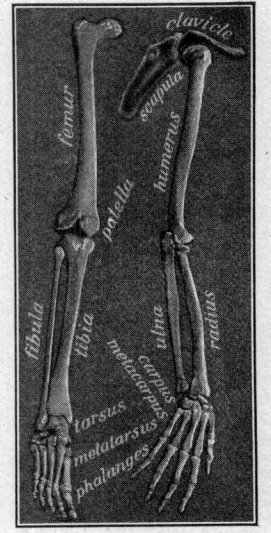

FIG. 92.—Bones of the leg at the left, and those of the arm at the right.

fibula, reaches from the knee to the ankle. The wrist bones, called *carpus,* are eight in number, while there are seven bones named *tarsus* forming the ankle. A single bone of the wrist is called a *carpal,* and one of the ankle bones is a *tarsal.*

Five bones are present in the palm of the hand, and the same number of bones are in the same part of the foot. There are three bones in each finger, and two in the thumb. There are also three bones present in each toe, except the great one which has only two.

Structure of Bone.—Bone is made hard by salts of lime, but there are many soft living cells in the bone. By placing a bone, such as a rib of any animal, in strong vinegar or other weak acid, the lime salts may be eaten out. Within a week the bone will become as elastic as a green willow twig.

Numerous channels extend through the bones for the purpose of lodging the nerves and blood vessels. The surface of bones is made of hard *compact bone,* while within is loose *spongy bone.* The ends of the long bones are nearly all spongy bone, while in the middle part is a cavity filled with soft white marrow. This gives lightness and much surface for the attachment of muscles.

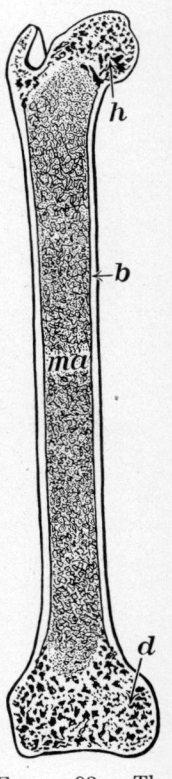

FIG. 93.—The thigh bone cut through the middle. *b,* hard bone; *h* and *d,* spongy bone; *ma,* marrow.

Every bone is covered on the outside with a tough membrane called *periosteum*. This serves for the attachment of the ends of muscles. It is also able to grow new bone to take the place of that which may be destroyed.

How the Bones Grow.—Most of the bones are at first in the form of a gristle called *cartilage*. This may be easily bent and pressed out of shape. In the young child, since much of the cartilage is not yet changed into bone, the legs may become bent or bowed if it is allowed to stand too much. Even children of school age sometimes make the bones grow into a bad shape by sitting on seats so high that the feet cannot touch the floor, or by leaning over the desk so as to cause round shoulders. Everyone should form the habit of sitting up straight, of keeping the shoulders held back in walking and the neck pressed back against the collar.

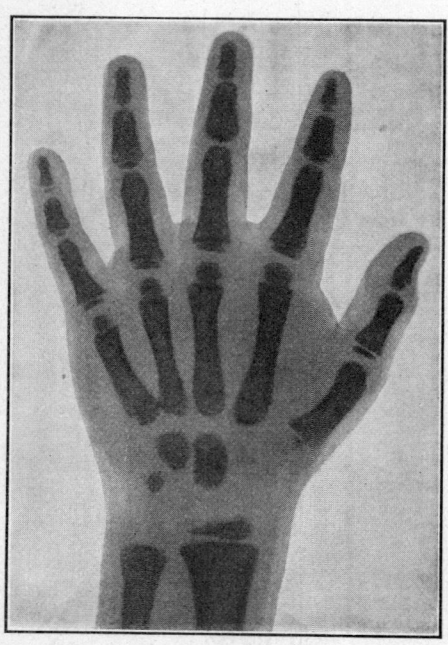

Fig. 94.—The bones in the hand of a child of five years. Only three of the eight wrist bones are formed and loose ends are seen on other bones. From an X-ray photograph.

Broken Bones.—A break in a bone is called a *fracture*. As the bones of children bend easily, they are seldom broken off completely, but are cracked somewhat like a tough stick when bent. Such an injury is known as a *green-stick fracture*. When the bone of an older person is broken, the ends usually sep-

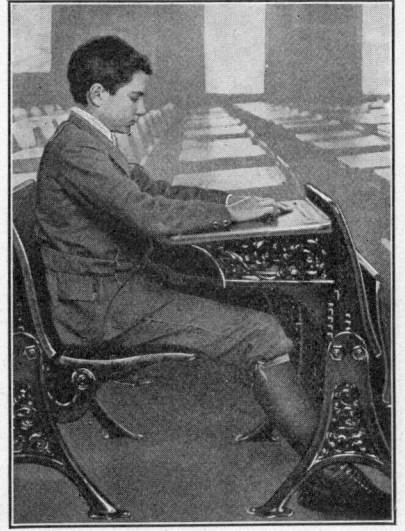

FIG. 95.—Proper position in school to prevent round shoulders.

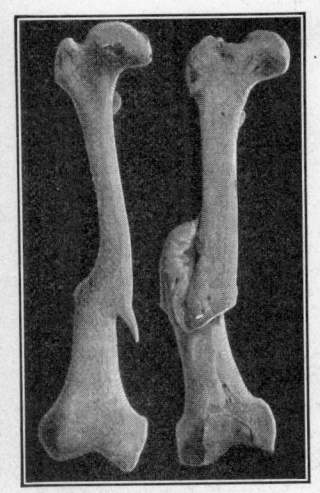

FIG. 96.—Thigh bones grown together after being broken. The one on the right was not properly cared for.

arate a little owing to the pull of the muscles. In order to set the bone properly the two ends must be brought together and held firmly in place by a thin board or sheet of metal bandaged on the limb.

First Care of a Broken Bone. —No one but a good surgeon is able to set a broken bone successfully. However, if a person with a fracture must be moved from the place of accident,

140 THE BONES

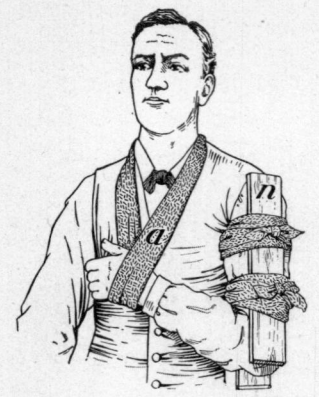

FIG. 97.—The way to hold the broken bone of the arm in place until the doctor comes.

it is wise to hold the broken bones in place by binding firmly on either side of the fracture, wrapped in clean cloth, a narrow board or flat stick.

In young persons, broken bones usually knit together in three or four weeks, but in persons over sixty years of age, healing may require several months.

The Joints.—The juncture of two or more bones is a *joint*, or *articulation*. The two general kinds of joints are the *movable* and the *immovable*. The immovable joints occur between the bones of the skull. The two important kinds of movable joints are the *ball and socket joint*, like that at the shoulder and hip, and the *hinge joint*, as seen at the knee and elbow.

In the movable joints, the ends of the bones are covered with a thin pad of gristle. Several tough bands of white stringy tissue called *ligaments* hold the bones in place and form a covering for the joint. This covering

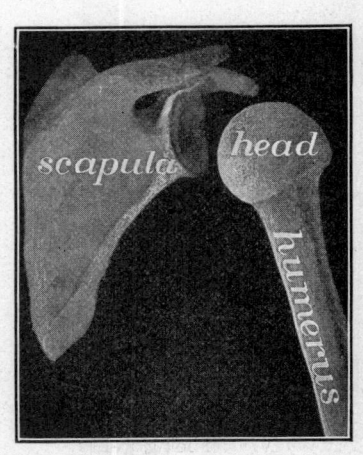

FIG. 98.—Ball and socket joint at the shoulder.

is lined with a tender membrane. It forms a thick fluid, like the white of egg. This is used to keep the joint moist and in smooth working condition.

Strain and Sprain.—By bending a joint too far or pushing the end of a bone to one side, the ligaments may be stretched or even torn. This results in swelling and tenderness called a *strain*.

A severe strain is a *sprain*. The best treatment to give at once, is to place the injured part in hot water or wrap it in cloths wrung out of very hot water, and change them every few minutes. At the end of a half-hour, the joint should be massaged by rubbing it toward the body, in order to move the collected lymph away to the veins. Unless the ligaments are torn, complete rest is not so helpful as careful exercise and frequent massaging.

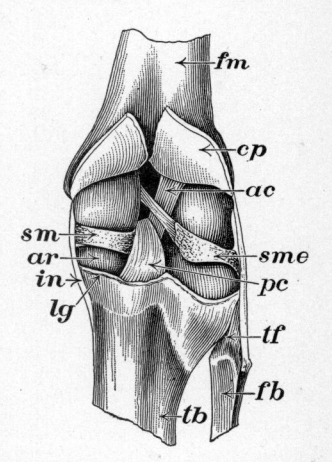

FIG. 99.—A knee joint cut open from behind to show the ligaments. *cp*, ligament cut off at *lg*.

Dislocation of Bones.—When at a joint, the end of one bone is forced backward, forward or to one side of the other bone, so far that it does not slip back into place, it is said to be *dislocated*. The ligaments may be somewhat torn or stretched. The patient should be placed in an easy position and a physician sent for at once, as the parts become very sore in a few hours. The bones at the knee and shoulder joints are the ones most frequently dislocated.

Effect of Alcohol and Other Narcotics on the Bones.— The blood furnishes the material out of which the bones are made. The blood receives its food for the body from the digestive system. The digestive system works properly only when the nervous system, which governs it, is in good condition. Tobacco, alcoholic drinks, and other narcotics are known to affect seriously the nervous, digestive and circulatory systems.

The organs removing the poisonous waste from the growing bones are often made unfit to perform their duties properly by the continued use of narcotics, especially those containing alcohol. This unremoved waste then affects the growing bones by slowing the living action of the cells. In many young persons, using much tobacco, the bones grow about one fourth slower than in healthy boys and girls. This fact has been clearly proved by many careful measurements of normal healthy boys, and those using tobacco regularly.

Practical Questions

1. Of what use are the bones? 2. Give the three parts of the skeleton. 3. Name the bones in the arm and forearm. 4. Name the bones of the leg. 5. How many bones in each toe and finger? 6. Name the bones on the side of the head. 7. Of what is bone made? 8. What is the periosteum? 9. Why should you sit and walk erect? 10. What is a fracture? 11. Describe the first care to be given a broken bone. 12. Name three kinds of joints. 13. Which joints allow motion in more than two directions? 14. What is a ligament? 15. What is a sprain?

CHAPTER XV

THE MUSCLES AND EXERCISE

The Muscles Forming the Lean Meat.—The rich red meat, called beefsteak, is made of muscle. The muscle of a person looks just like the muscle of a cow. All lean meat is muscle. With the exception of the bones, skin, and digestive organs, the body is composed chiefly of muscle, with blood vessels and nerves running through it. This muscle substance is not one undivided mass, but is made of about 500 distinct parts, each of which is known as a *muscle*.

The Nature of a Muscle.—A muscle is made of fine threads called *fibers*. These are held together by a fine, web like connecting tissue. The muscle fibers are made to shorten and thicken by an order sent to them through the nerves. When the fibers become shorter this makes the whole muscle shorter. The shortening of a muscle is *contraction* and the lengthening of it is known as the *relaxing*.

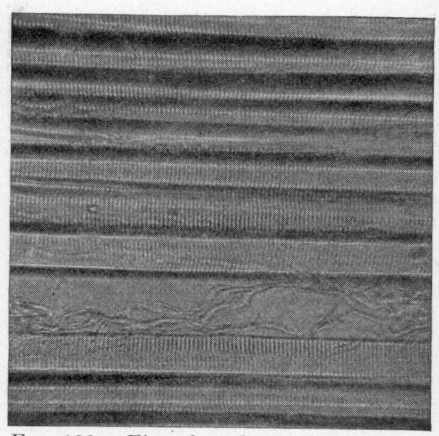

FIG. 100.—Fine threads of fibers forming a muscle. Much enlarged.

144 MUSCLES AND EXERCISE

When a muscle has one end fixed at the shoulder and the other end fastened to a bone of

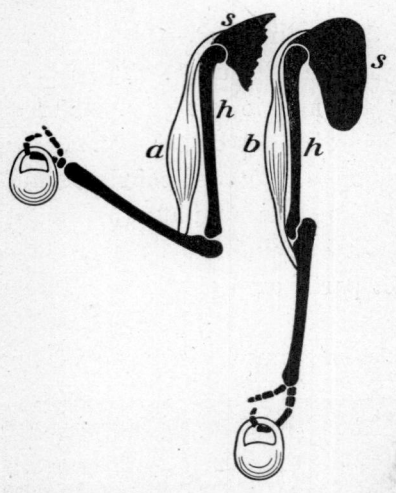

Fig. 101.—Showing how the muscle thickens when it shortens to draw up the arm. *a* and *b*, muscle. The bones are in black.

the forearm the shortening or contraction of the muscle pulls the forearm upward. In a similar way, the movements of the fingers, legs and toes are produced by the contraction of various muscles.

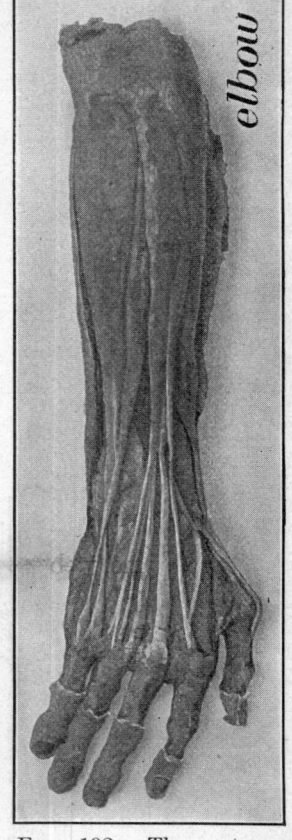

Fig. 102.— The extensor muscles on the back of the forearm. Note the tendons at the wrist. From a photograph.

Arrangement of Muscles.— Both ends of a muscle are not attached to the same bone, but each end is fixed to a different bone, so that a contraction of the muscle must move one of the bones. So some of the muscles extend from the humerus to the fingers, and others from the hip bone to below the knee.

The muscles act like levers. That is one part of the bone, usually the end or a place near the end, is held fast in a joint, while the muscle is fixed to another part. The *triceps muscle* is fixed to the elbow end of the ulna, and pulls it up so as to force the other end down, as when one strikes the hand on the table. Pulling on the *biceps muscle* attached in front of the elbow brings the forearm up. Notice that this muscle grows thicker as it shortens.

Very often the muscle fibers are not fixed directly to the bone, but to a cord of tough white fibers, called a *tendon* which is joined to the bone. The hard cords felt in the wrist, when the fingers are moved, are tendons. On the back of the hand, three or four tendons may also be felt, and the skin seen to be pushed out by them when the fingers are worked. The largest is the *tendon of Achilles*, attached to the heel bone.

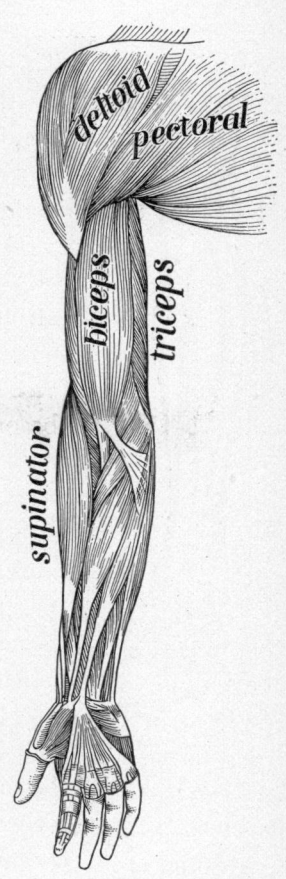

FIG. 103.—Muscles on the front of the arm. Note the white cords, the tendons at the wrist.

Kinds of Muscles.—The muscles forming the lean meat are called *voluntary muscles*, because one can move them whenever he wishes. Another set of muscles is named *involuntary*, because the will has no control over them. These muscles help form the walls of nearly all tubes in the body. They regulate the size of the blood vessels and cause the movements of the stomach and the intestines.

The *involuntary muscles* are made of short, spindle shaped cells. The alcohol drinker cannot prevent the lengthening of these muscles in the blood vessels of the skin, causing it to become red. No one can prevent the movement of these muscles in the stomach after food enters, nor can one stop the beating of the heart. These muscles are made to act by a set of nerves called sympathetic, which do not obey our will.

Kinds of Voluntary Muscles.—There are two chief kinds of voluntary muscles. One kind is called *flexor muscles* because they bend a limb, while the other is known as *extensor muscles* because they straighten a limb. Several flexor muscles lie on the palm side of the hand and arm, and also on the back of the leg. Important extensor muscles lie on the back of the hand and arm, and on the

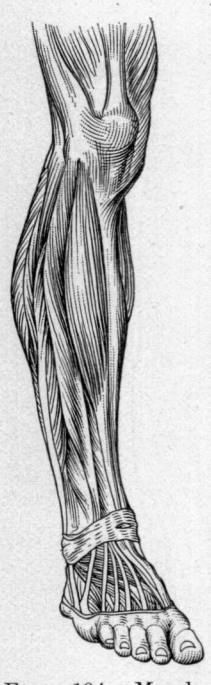

FIG. 104.—Muscles of the leg showing how they pass into tendons at the ankle.

MUSCLES AND EXERCISE

front of the leg. Flexor muscles bend the fingers, arms, legs, and toes, and extensor muscles pull them straight.

Muscles of Expression.—The score of muscles controlling the eyes, mouth and other features of the face are the muscles of expression. On their action depends largely whether one has a pleasing or ugly countenance. In one who is accustomed to pout, frown or cry about every trifle or annoyance, the muscles become so trained to pulling down the corners of the mouth, pushing out the lips, and wrinkling the forehead, that the face can never have a pleasant look.

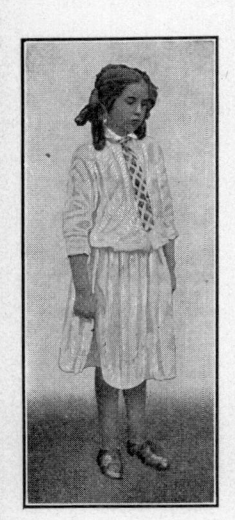

FIG. 105.—Using the pouting muscles.

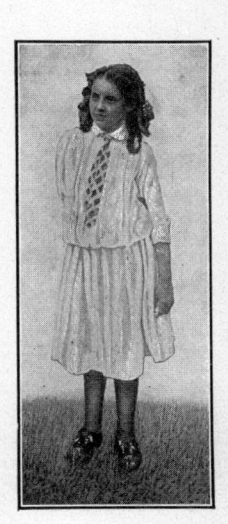

FIG. 106.—Using the muscles for a pleasant expression.

Need of Exercise.—To exercise the muscles means to use them. No boy or girl can have a strong, well formed body unless the muscles are exercised. Every time a muscle is moved, the vessels in it enlarge and allow more blood to flow with the food to make the muscle grow.

Exercise is also of great service in pressing the lymph with its waste matter out of its chinks and crevices into the lymph channels. The pressure of the muscles as they contract, squeezes on the lymph and blood vessels, so as to help the circulation. Since the whole body has its waste carried away and an abundance of life-giving oxygen supplied by exercise, one always feels better after a vigorous walk or the playing of an outdoor game.

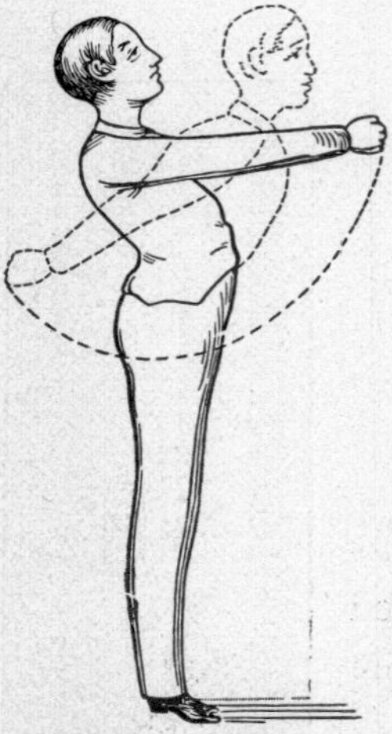

How to Exercise.—Since nearly every one is obliged to do some walking, certain muscles of the legs are sure to get some exercise. In ordinary walking, however, less than one half of the hundred muscles in the legs are brought into use. To get the best exercise out of walking one must walk as fast as possible, and let the arms swing to and fro at the sides. The chin should be held in, the chest pushed out, and the neck thrown back against the collar.

FIG. 107.—One way to exercise.

A regular period of one or two hours should be devoted to exercise every day. Boys and girls who live on the farm or have gardens to care for, may bring into use nearly all the muscles in attending to the various duties about the home. The muscles least likely to get the proper exercise and the ones needing it most are those of the chest.

Cause of Round Shoulders and Flat Chests.—The lungs cannot be kept strong and healthy without being fully expanded. There must be plenty of space in the chest cavity to let them expand. The size of the chest will depend upon the exercise of the lungs and the muscles of the chest. Very few duties in life call these muscles into vigorous use. They are, therefore, often weak and when one sits down they permit the shoulders to droop, the head to bend forward, and the chest to be pushed inward. Even in standing a similar position is often taken.

Preventing Round Shoulders and Flat Chests.—Weak lungs can often be avoided, and many of the quarter-million deaths in this country from lung diseases

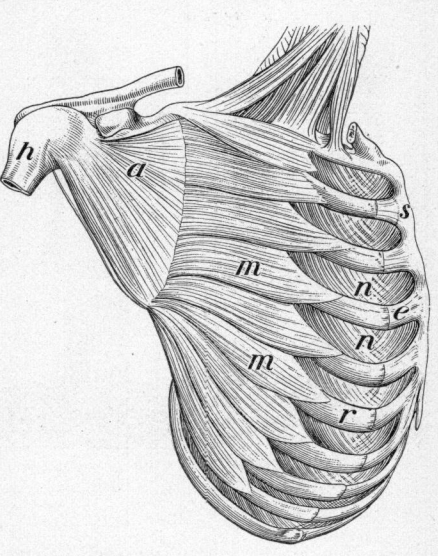

FIG. 108.—The chest muscles which need exercise to strengthen the lungs. *r*, rib; *s*, breastbone; *m*, and *n*, important muscles in breathing.

prevented by proper exercise. The practice of taking in full breaths, for a few minutes each day, when out in the open air should become a habit. This enlarges the chest. This exercise will be still more effective if, while the lungs are full of air, the chest is beat lightly with the hand. Ten or fifteen minutes daily should be spent in swinging the arms upward and downward, and forward, outward and backward until the hands meet in front and behind the back.

Forming the habit of sitting erect at a table or desk, and of walking with the shoulders well thrown back will do much to develop a well-formed body and promote health.

The Best Games for Exercise.—Exercise can do much more than medicine to give good health. It is almost as important to play as to work. Games like cards, checkers and dominoes may help to keep boys and

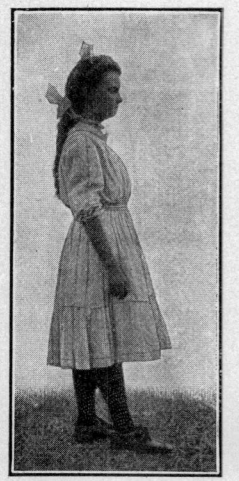

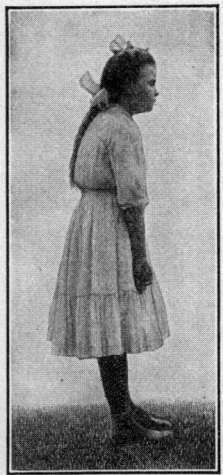

FIG. 109. Graceful and ungraceful attitudes in standing. The latter causes round shoulders and weak lungs.

girls, and even older persons, out of mischief, but they do not make the body strong and ready for the great work of life like games played in the open air, calling into use the muscles.

Swimming, rowing and running are excellent forms of exercise, but they must not be carried to excess. Baseball, shinny and skating are also splendid games for bringing into use many muscles. Tennis, however, is the best game of all for exercising the largest number of muscles, and especially those of the chest. When games cannot be played in the open air, the gymnasium offers many helpful forms of exercise which both boys and girls should use in helping to build strong bodies and insure long life and health.

Tobacco and the Muscles.—Nicotine causes the involuntary muscles of the small blood vessels to contract, and thus shut off some of the nourishment intended for the growth of the muscles. The habitual use of tobacco affects the growth of the young in a very marked degree.

At Yale College during four years the non-users of tobacco gained one fourth more in height, and in the girth of the chest, than the habitual users of tobacco. Doctor Seaver, of New Haven, found on examining a large number of young men, that the tobacco users at 18 years of age were not so large and well developed as the non-users only 17 years old. These facts show that the use of much tobacco, either by smoking or chewing, is quite certain to hinder the full growth of the muscles.

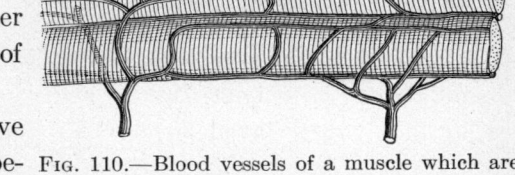

Those who have had much experience with boys

FIG. 110.—Blood vessels of a muscle which are affected by much use of tobacco.

say that smokers are not able to control their muscles accurately, and that they can discover the tobacco users by noting the trembling of the hand when they try to hold it perfectly still or attempt to draw a straight line.

How Alcohol Affects the Muscles.—Alcohol may stimulate the muscles for a few minutes, somewhat in the same way that a whip urges forward a horse, but recent experiments all agree in showing that the daily amount of work accomplished by men using alcohol is always less than that done by the total abstainers. On this account no athlete while in training makes use of whisky, wine or beer. Soldiers on forced marches are found to make better progress when denied the use of alcohol and given beef tea. Brigadier General A. W. Greely says it should be strongly urged that no alcoholic drink be used by soldiers undergoing great physical hardship and continued exhausting labor.

Practical Questions

1. What is a muscle? 2. Of what is a muscle made? 3. Tell something about the arrangement of muscles. 4. What is a tendon? 5. What action has a muscle? 6. Name two kinds of muscles. 7. Where are the involuntary muscles found? 8. Where are the extensor muscles on the arm? 9. What is the use of flexor muscles? 10. What makes a muscle become strong? 11. Why does exercise make one feel good? 12. Why do many persons have round shoulders? 13. How may flat chests be prevented? 14. Name some good forms of exercise. 15. Give facts showing that tobacco injures muscles. 16. What shows that alcohol does not help the muscles do good work?

Suggestions for the Teacher

During the study of this Chapter, a special effort should be made by the pupils to learn how to stand properly and walk gracefully. A few minutes daily exercise directed by the teacher will do much to correct the drooping shoulders and awkward shuffling gait common to many school children.

CHAPTER XVI

HOW THE BODY IS GOVERNED

Need of a Manager.—There are over five hundred separate organs in the body, each having a distinct duty to perform. Every muscle and every gland has a special work, but all the organs must act together in harmony to keep the body in health. For accomplishing this a general manager is needed to direct the work. This manager is the nervous system, which tells each organ when to act and how much work to do.

If there were no nervous system, the muscles could not be made to move the body, or the stomach to digest the food. When one takes a bite of food an order comes by the nerves to the salivary glands to make saliva and send it out into the mouth. A moment later other orders are given for digestive juices to flow into the stomach. Thus the right work is done at the right time and in the right place by the manager's command.

Parts of the Nervous System.—The nervous system is made of three parts: 1. The *brain,* located in the skull; 2. the *spinal cord*, hanging in the inch-wide canal of the spinal column; 3. the *nerves* which appear like white cords extending from the brain and spinal cord outward as they divide into finer branches throughout the body. The brain and spinal cord give orders and the nerves carry these orders to the organs (Fig. 111).

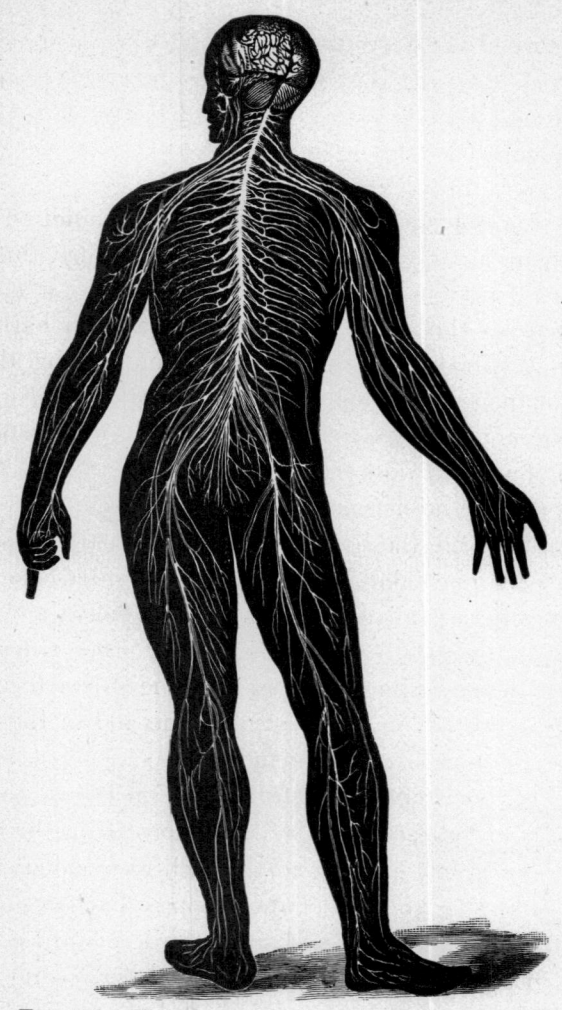

Fig. 111.—The nervous system viewed from behind

Structure of the Nervous System.—A slice cut across the brain or spinal cord shows that part of the nerve substance is white and part is gray. The gray matter is made of tiny irregular masses called *cell bodies,* while the white matter is formed of fine threads named nerve fibers. These fibers are fastened to the cell bodies and are, therefore, true parts of them.

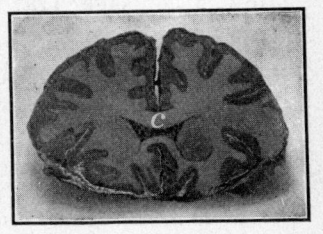

A complete *nerve cell* consists of a cell body with from two to a dozen fine threads called *processes* extending out from it. One of these processes is often from one to three feet in length. This long process is a *nerve fiber.* A bundle of nerve fibers forms a *nerve.*

FIG. 112.—A slice across the brain to show white and gray matter.

The Nerves.—The bodies of the nerve cells are all located in the brain or spinal cord, or very near to these two parts. From these cell bodies, the processes extend to the face, the arms and the legs. Thousands of these processes at the under surface of the brain and along the spinal cord are collected into many bundles to form the nerves (Fig. 115).

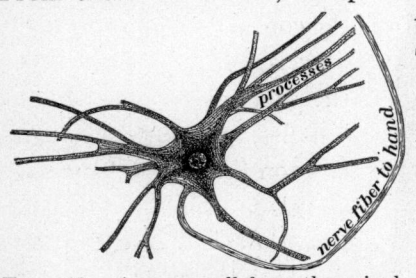

FIG. 113.—A nerve cell from the spinal cord. Much enlarged.

The nerves connected with the brain are called *cranial nerves.* They pass through holes in the floor of the skull. The *spinal nerves* are those joined to the spinal cord. A third set of nerves, branching throughout the body from some bunches of cell bodies along the front side of the backbone, are named *sympathetic nerves* (Fig. 117).

How a Message Travels on a Nerve.—There are two chief kinds of nerves. One kind called *sending nerves* carry messages from the brain and cord to the muscles and other organs to make them act. Another kind, known as the *receiving nerves*, carry messages of seeing, hearing and feeling from various parts of the body to the spinal cord and brain. The message telling that the finger is burnt or that an apple is sweet travels on a receiving nerve.

Sometimes receiving nerve fibers and sending nerve fibers are bound together in the same bundle as in the spinal nerves. Messages may then travel side by side but in opposite directions as when a baseball is caught. The feeling of the ball as it touches the hand rushes up the receiving nerve fibers to the cord, which quick as lightning sends a message down the sending nerve fibers to the muscles, making the hand close on the ball. A message travels so rapidly on a nerve that the news of a hurt toe can reach the brain in one half the time between two ticks of a watch.

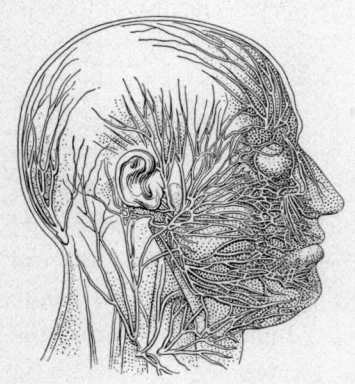

FIG. 114.—Some of the nerves of the face.

The Cranial Nerves.—There are twelve pairs of cranial

nerves joined to the base of the brain. One pair, the olfactory, extends to the nose, four pairs to the eyes, and one pair to the ears. The others are distributed to the head, neck and shoulders, with the exception of one pair which goes to the lungs and stomach.

The Spinal Nerves.—There are 31 pairs of nerves joined to the spinal cord. Each of these nerves is united to the cord by two branches. The front one is called the *sending root* because the messages sent by the brain or cord to make an organ act pass through this root. The back branch is named the *receiving root* as all news of heat, cold, pain and pressure pass through this root.

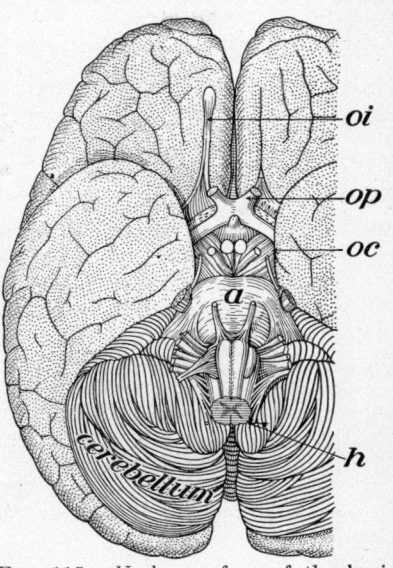

FIG. 115.—Under surface of the brain showing stumps of nerves cut off. *oi*, nerve of smell; *op*, nerve of sight; *h*, spinal cord cut off at the medulla.

Some of the spinal nerves such as those supplying the arms and legs are two or three feet long. The *great sciatic nerve*, which is nearly as large as a lead pencil and extends down the back of the leg, is the largest nerve in the body.

The Sympathetic Nerves.—On either side of the backbone, and within the body cavity, is a chain of bunches of nerve cells. Several other similar bunches lie near the stomach and also lower down in the body cavity. These bunches of nerve cells are called *ganglia*. These ganglia with the nerve fibers joining them and extending from

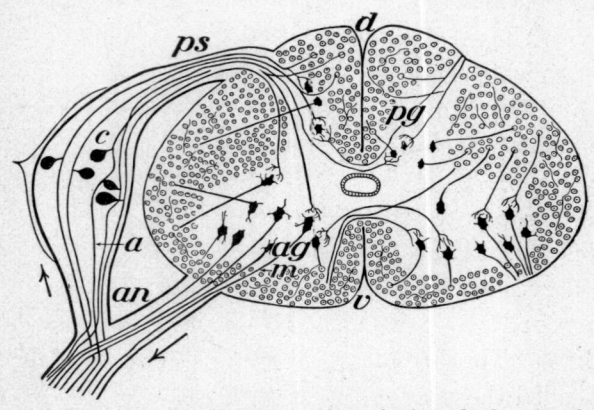

FIG. 116.—Diagram of a slice across the spinal cord, showing the roots of a spinal nerve to the arm on the left. The arrows show which way the messages travel. The little circles are the cut ends of fibers extending up and down the cord. Only a few of the thousands of fibers really present are here shown.

them to the glands and involuntary muscles all over the body, form the *sympathetic nervous system* (Fig. 117).

Use of the Sympathetic Nervous System.—The nerves of the sympathetic system supply the stomach, intestines, liver, pancreas, heart, lungs, and the muscles in the veins and arteries in all regions of the body. This system acts without our knowledge and cannot be controlled by our wishes. When food goes into the stomach, a message is received by the sympathetic system to make the gastric glands give out juice to digest the food. When, by running, we use up the oxygen in the muscles, it is the sympathetic system that tells the heart to beat faster and send more blood bearing the oxygen for the hungry tissues. When we are hot, the sympathetic system orders the sweat glands to give out sweat to cool the body.

The Spinal Cord.—This consists of a bundle of nerve fibers inclosing a column of cell bodies. The outer part of the cord therefore appears white, while the central H-shaped part is gray. The cord is about eighteen inches long and as large in diameter as the little finger. It is joined by 31 pairs of nerves which extend to all parts of the body, except the head.

The spinal cord has two uses. It conducts messages between the brain and the nerves of the arms, legs and trunk. It also acts independently of the brain and causes many of the muscular movements such as are required in walking thoughtlessly or in withdrawing the

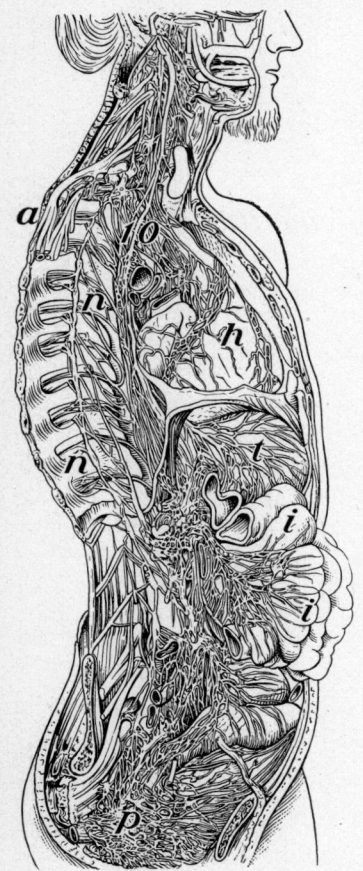

Fig. 117.—Part of the sympathetic nervous system seen from the side. *n*, one of the two chief cords; *t*, *i*, and *p*, branches to the organs.

finger or foot from a sharp tack or burning object. Such performances are spoken of as *reflex action*.

Reflex Action.—This is any action of the nervous system without the use of the will. Tickling the foot of the

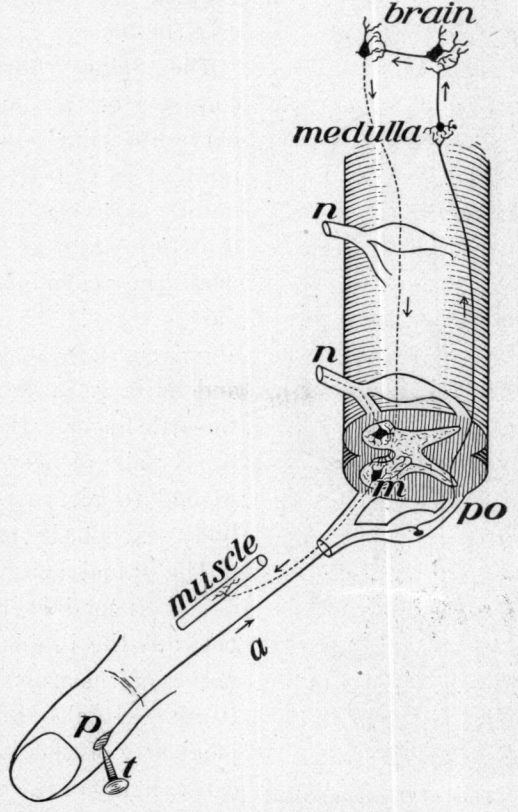

FIG. 118.—How reflex action occurs. The pain caused by the tack *t*, goes up the fiber *a*, and shifts off to the cell *m* which sends a message down from the muscle to move and draw away the finger. The message may also go up to the brain and down as shown.

soundest sleeper causes it to be moved, but the brain was asleep and did not act. The cell bodies in the cord aroused by the tickling sent a message to make the muscles move. The squirming of a snake with a mashed head, the jumping of a chicken with its head cut off, and the wriggling of the pieces of a freshly cleaned eel, placed in the hot frying pan, are reflex acts in which the brain has no part.

Reflex action causes the hand stuck with a pin to be withdrawn before the brain can act. The pain travels up the nerve fiber of the arm and around through the spinal cord, exciting the cell bodies there to send a message out to the muscles to withdraw the arm. A fraction of a second later the brain feels the pain. The beating of the heart, breathing, the movements of the stomach or any other activity caused by the sympathetic system is reflex action.

The Brain.—The brain almost completely fills the cavity of the cranium. The three main parts are: the *cerebrum* or *great brain*, the *cerebellum* or *little brain* and the *medulla oblongata* or *stem* of the brain, which joins the spinal cord.

The brain, like the spinal cord, is made of both white and gray matter. That is, there are millions of cell bodies with their processes or nerve fibers extending from them and forming a thick, irregular network. The gray matter of the brain is largely on the outside, where it forms a layer an eighth of an inch thick, called the *cortex* (Fig. 112).

The Cerebrum or Great Brain.—This composes seven eighths of the entire brain. It is divided into halves, named hemispheres, by a deep cleft, the *longitudinal fissure*, extending from before, backward. The surface of the cerebrum is very uneven, as there are many folds separated by grooves an inch deep. The folds are known as *convolutions*. They are for the purpose of giving a greater extent to the cortex on which intelligence in animal life in general depends. Fish, frogs, snakes, and birds have no folds in their cerebrum, while rabbits and cats have very few folds. In horses and monkeys, the cerebrum has many folds, but the number is less than in man.

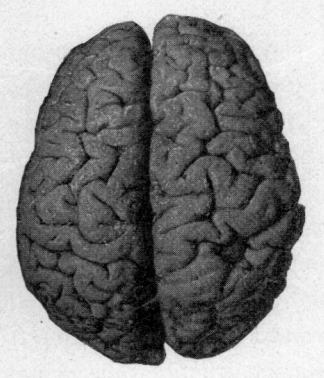

FIG. 119.—The upper surface of the brain showing the hemispheres and folds. From a photograph.

Use of the Cerebrum.—The cerebrum is the seat of the mind. It is the thinking organ. Different portions of it have different duties to perform. The middle part of the cortex is concerned in receiving the messages from the nerves of feeling and in directing the movements of the muscles. The back part is used in seeing, and the part near the ear for hearing. The front part of the cortex,

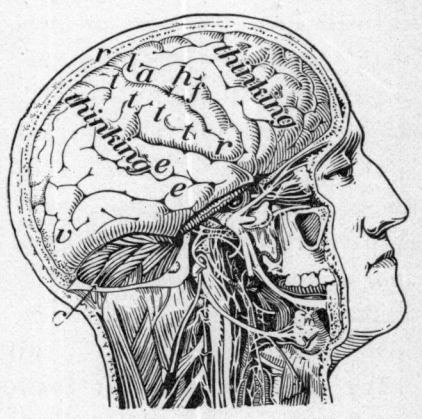

FIG. 120.—Right half of the skull cut away to show the brain. *c*, cerebellum; *l*, *a*, *h*, and *f*, part of the cerebrum used in moving muscles; *t*, used in feeling; *e*, used in hearing; *v*, used in seeing.

and some other portions of it, help us to think, but how it is done no one knows.

Many nerve fibers connect the cerebrum with the other parts of the brain and with the spinal cord. Most of the nerve fibers from the right side of the cerebrum cross to the opposite side in the stem of the brain, so as to connect with the left half of the spinal cord. In this way the muscles on the left side of the body are controlled by the right half of the brain. Likewise the muscles on the right side of the body are moved by the left half of the brain.

The Cerebellum or Little Brain and Medulla Oblongata.—The cerebellum lies beneath the hind part of the cerebrum. It has many deep cuts and folds on its surface. Its use is not well understood. It is connected with the spinal cord and the other parts of the brain by three bands of nerve fibers on each side. Animals in which it is injured can move the muscles, but they cannot make them work together properly. As a result they tumble about like a drunken man.

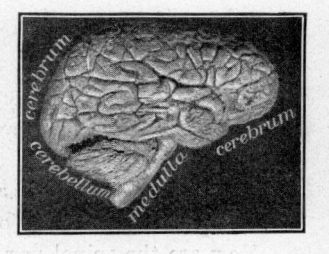

FIG. 121.—The brain from the side. From a photograph.

The *medulla oblongata* is the *stem of the brain* connecting it with a cord. It is the only portion of the brain whose destruction causes immediate death. The cell bodies in the medulla control the breathing and the heart beat, and also have much to do with the action of the alimentary canal.

Paralysis and Apoplexy.—Paralysis is lack of power to

move the muscles or lack of feeling in any part of the skin. It is caused by an injury to the nerve fibers, or to the cell bodies. If a nerve in the arm is cut or pressed upon hard, the muscle to which it extends cannot be moved. Pressing upon the nerve of the leg sometimes puts the foot to sleep. A pressure of a bone on the spinal cord may cause paralysis.

Paralysis which affects one side of the body may be caused by the clogging of a blood vessel in the brain or the breaking of such a vessel. The blood runs out and forms a clot, which presses on the cell bodies or their fibers which carry messages to move the muscles. When paralysis comes on suddenly and causes unconsciousness it is called *apoplexy*.

Practical Questions

1. Of what use is the nervous system? 2. Name the three parts of the nervous system. 3. Of what is the gray nerve matter made? 4. What is the form of a complete nerve cell? 5. Of what does a nerve consist? 6. What are the cranial nerves? 7. What are the spinal nerves? 8. How does a sending nerve differ from a receiving nerve? 9. Name some regions supplied by the cranial nerves. 10. How are the spinal nerves joined to the cord? 11. What is supplied by the sympathetic nervous system? 12. Explain how the sympathetic nervous system acts. 13. Describe the spinal cord. 14. Give the uses of the spinal cord. 15. Explain reflex action. 16. Give the parts of the brain. 17. What is the cortex? 18. Describe the cerebrum. 19. What is the use of the cerebrum? 20. Why does the left side of the cerebrum control muscles on the right side of the body? 21. Of what use is the cerebellum? 22. Give some facts about the medulla. 23. What is paralysis? 24. What causes paralysis? 25. What is apoplexy?

CHAPTER XVII

THE CARE OF THE NERVOUS SYSTEM AND HOW NARCOTICS AFFECT IT

The Brain and the Mind.—The brain is smaller in women than in men, because the body is smaller. The brain of a man weighs about three pounds, and that of a woman weighs three or four ounces less. A good mind does not depend so much upon the size of the brain as upon the size and number of the processes of the nerve cells. An ox of 2000 pounds has a smaller brain than a man weighing 120 pounds. The brain of a whale weighing 10,000 pounds is no heavier than the brain of some men. The human brain is 1-44 the weight of the body, while that of an elephant is 1-500 the weight of its body.

Why the Brain Needs Exercise.—In teachers, lawyers and business men, who do much thinking, the brain continues to grow until near the fortieth year of age, but in those who shovel coal or do the same work day after day requiring no thinking, the brain stops growing after the twentieth year of age. A muscle grows by use and the same is true of the brain. One cannot use the mind without using the brain.

How to Exercise the Brain.—In the young there are many nerve cells with short processes. These may be made to grow by using the cells, as when one studies. Thinking causes the blood to flow to the brain and thus bring more nourishment for the cells. Memorizing the words of a book does not exercise the brain so much, as thinking out what the words mean and then trying to put the thought into one's own language.

The brain upon which the mind depends grows faster in youth than it does later in life. If the mind is not developed when one is young, it can never become as strong as it otherwise would by work in later years. On this account one should attend school regularly and try faithfully to master his lessons while young.

How Habits are Formed.—The doing of one thing over and over again calls into action the same set of nerve cells, and they finally become so accustomed to act, that they do so without the aid of the will, and often even against it. This is *habit*. A boy long accustomed to swearing, acting rudely, eating rapidly, or looking sullen cannot refrain from these ungentlemanly habits later in life, even when honestly trying to do so. The cultivation of agreeable manners and pleasant looks not only makes friends in school, but success in later life.

The Danger of Bad Thoughts.—Evil thoughts passing often through the nerve cells leave a blot there which can never be entirely erased. The first step toward wrong doing is in wrong thinking. Many cases are known where the reading of books and newspapers describing wicked acts has affected the nerve cells so as to cause the reader to commit robbery and other crimes.

The youth who causes to pass through his nervous system into his mind noble thoughts from good people and good books, and who learns industry, patience and politeness, is sure of friends and success in life. The mind is like a piece of ground which if not sowed with good seed and cultivated, will grow up with worthless weeds. It is, therefore, important that one should keep in good company and think and talk about what will make life more pleasant and useful.

Sleep.—It is just as important to rest as to work. The only time when the nervous system rests completely is during sleep. Grown persons, as a rule, should sleep eight hours every night, while those younger should add ten or fifteen minutes for every year under the age of twenty.

Continued loss of sleep is sure to result in ill health sooner or later. The time for retiring should be the same every night, so that one will drop off to sleep within five minutes after lying down. Hard thinking or excited talking just before going to bed is likely to keep one awake.

Without the advice of a physician medicine should never be taken to make one sleep. Babies should never be given drops to put them to sleep. Drinking a half cup of hot milk, placing the feet in hot water a few minutes, or taking a warm bath is an aid to sleep. One or more windows of the bedroom should be open both at the top and bottom to admit plenty of fresh air.

The Nervous System and Tobacco.—Tobacco habitually used by the young has a more serious effect on the nervous system than on any other part of the body. It prevents the brain cells from developing to their full extent and results in a slow and dull mind.

Chief Justice Brewer of the United States Supreme

168 NERVOUS SYSTEM—HOW NARCOTICS AFFECT IT

Court says: "No cigarette smoker can attain the highest position in the world." At Harvard during fifty years, no habitual user of tobacco ever graduated at the head of his class. The New York Division of the Reading Railroad,

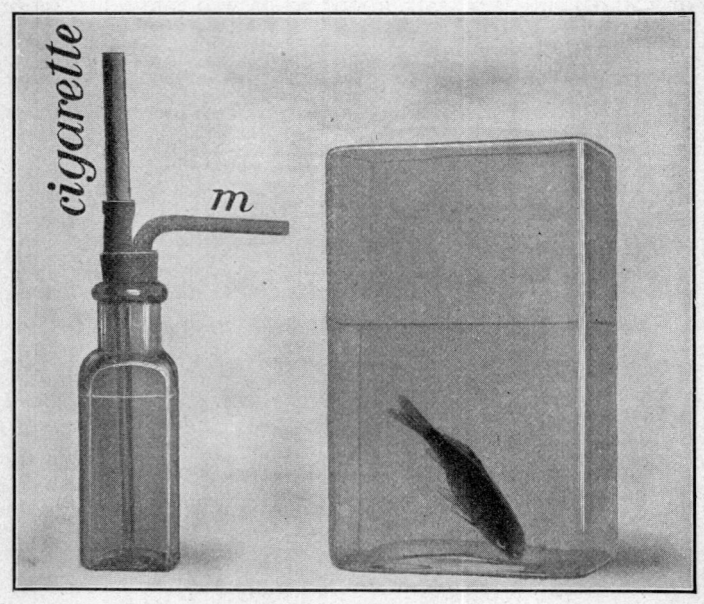

FIG. 122.—Experiment to show how tobacco affects the nerves. *m* is a tube through which the air is sucked from the bottle nearly full of water. This draws the smoke from the burning cigarette through the tube down into the water. The poison in the smoke from six cigarettes was caught in the water which when poured into the jar with the fish put it to sleep in a half hour and later killed it.

which prohibits cigarette smoking by employees, says: "Men who smoke cigarettes are liable to lapses of memory, and it is not safe to trust the lives of passengers in the hands of men who have that failing."

How Cigarettes Affect the Minds of Boys.—Long and careful observations by many persons show that cigarette smoking, not only clouds the intellect of the young, but also tends to make criminals of them. Doctor Hutchison, of the Kansas State Reformatory, says: "Cigarettes are the cause of the downfall of more of the inmates of this institution than all other vicious habits combined." Of 4117 boys received into the Illinois State Reformatory, 4000 were in the habit of using tobacco, and over 3000 were cigarette smokers.

It is unwise to begin the use of tobacco, because when the habit is once acquired, it can be broken only by one with a strong mind, who is willing to endure suffering caused by the longing nerve cells for several weeks after deprived of their accustomed poison.

How Alcohol Affects the Brain.—Much of the alcoholic drink taken is absorbed by the blood vessels of the stomach, so that it reaches the nerve cells in a few minutes. A large amount of alcohol completely paralyzes them. A cupful of whisky will make a boy dead drunk and may kill him. This deathlike sleep will last for several hours, because the alcohol has numbed the cells of the brain so that it cannot act.

One or two tablespoonfuls of whisky, or a glass of wine, taken by a boy will make the hand unsteady and cause a tottering gait. This is because the alcohol partly stupefies the cells in the cerebellum, which in health make the muscles act in harmony. A drunken man reels and staggers when he has taken enough strong drink to prevent the cerebellum from doing its work.

Alcohol Makes the Nerves Unsteady.—The trembling of the hands when attempting to hold them perfectly quiet, and a lack of power to stand erect without any swaying of the body, are sometimes seen even in moderate drinkers. The country of Sweden in 1905 experimented with her soldiers, to learn whether alcohol helped them to shoot better. On several different days each man was given four tablespoonfuls of brandy, and they were then ordered to shoot at a mark. The result was that they hit the mark only two thirds as many times in 30 shots as upon the days when no brandy was given them. The trials were made under varying conditions several times a day, and the result was always the same.

Evil Effects of Alcohol as shown by Experiments on Animals.—The nervous system of a dog or cat is very similar to that of man, and is acted upon by drugs much in the same way as that of man. Alcohol given to dogs soon changes their character, even when the quantity fed them is small. They become timid, nervous, irritable and cross. They are so easily frightened that the sound of whistles and bells in the distance causes them to yelp and howl in an excited manner. Instead of responding to caresses they sometimes snap viciously at the hand put out to pet them.

Alcohol Makes the Nervous System Weak.—The continued use of alcohol, even in such light drinks as that of beer, is known to have a weakening effect on the nervous system and to render it more liable to disease. The persons most generally attacked by sunstroke and heat stroke are the users of alcoholic drinks.

Of 70 persons killed by sunstroke in recent years, it is known that all but seven used intoxicating drinks. The soldiers in Austria are not allowed to carry any brandy during warm weather.

Alcohol and the Mind.—Since the mind depends upon the brain and the health of its cells, it is reasonable to suppose that anything which has a bad effect upon the brain might also have a like effect on the mind. Experience shows that alcohol does harm the mind. Reports from many countries furnish the evidence that insanity, robbery and murder increase with the increased use of alcoholic drinks, and decrease wherever the law prevents the sale of liquor.

Alcohol Makes Persons Insane.—An insane person is said to be crazy or out of his mind. He cannot think or reason rightly and often does not know his own brothers and sisters. He must be cared for by others, and sometimes must be shut up in a place called an *asylum* to prevent him from harming himself or others.

The reports of the asylums in England and Wales show that about three thousand five hundred persons are every year made insane by the use of alcoholic drink. In Waterford County, Ireland, one in every 28 persons is a drunkard. As a consequence one in every 104 of the population is insane.

Alcohol Sends People to Prison.—After the terrible earthquake at San Francisco, in 1906, all of the saloons were ordered closed for fear that the drunken persons would hurt the homeless women and children. As a result, the number of arrests by the police were only from two to six per day, for several months, until the saloons were opened again. Then the arrests were from fifty to over one hundred daily, and it was necessary to put extra policemen on duty.

Inquiry has shown that of the 13,402 convicts in our prisons at one time, 4000 said that the first cause of their crime was alcohol.

Chloroform, Ether and Cocaine.—Chloroform and ether are great blessings to humanity, when rightly used, in preventing terrible suffering which would otherwise occur in performing operations on the human body. When the fumes of these drugs are breathed into the lungs they are carried by the blood to the nerve cells of the brain, and put them to sleep in a few minutes. This use of chloroform was discovered in 1846 by Doctor William Morton of Boston.

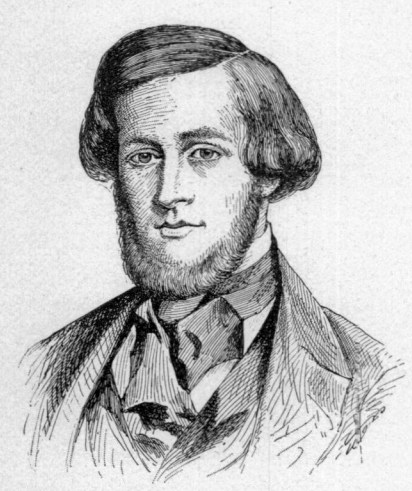

FIG. 123.—William Morton, who discovered the use of chloroform.

Cocaine deadens for a few minutes the feeling of the nerves wherever it is dropped on the skin or forced under the skin through a hollow needle. The dentists sometimes use it to prevent much pain in pulling a tooth. Chloroform, ether and cocaine are dangerous drugs, and should not be used by anyone except experienced persons. Because of the evil effects of the continual use of cocaine, a law was passed in 1908 forbidding the transmission by mail of any patent medicine containing cocaine.

Practical Questions

1. Give some facts about the weight of the brain. 2. Why should the brain have exercise? 3. How can you exercise your brain? 4. When does the brain grow most? 5. What is habit? 6. How is a habit formed? 7. Why is it wrong to harbor bad thoughts? 8. How much time should be given to sleep? 9. What may aid one in going to sleep? 10. How does tobacco affect the nervous system? 11. Why is it wrong for boys to smoke cigarettes? 12. Describe the effect of alcohol on the brain. 13. How does alcohol affect the nerves? 14. Give facts showing that alcohol makes the nervous system weak. 15. What shows that alcohol hurts the mind? 16. Give facts showing that alcohol makes persons insane. 17. Show that alcohol sends people to prison. 18. What effect have chloroform and ether on the body? 19. Who discovered the use of chloroform? 20. How does cocaine affect the nerves?

CHAPTER XVIII

ORGANS FOR RECEIVING KNOWLEDGE

How We Learn of Things About Us.—The organs for receiving knowledge of the things about us are called *sense organs*. They are to the nerves what the telephone transmitter is to the telephone wire. These sense organs are the endings of the receiving nerves. They are the means by which all news get on to the nerves to be carried to the spinal cord and brain.

One's knowledge of an apple is secured through certain sense organs in the skin touching the apple, through the sense organs in the nose catching the odor of the apple, through the sense organs in the tongue taking note of the sweetness, and through the sense organs of sight affected by the light coming from the apple. None of these impulses excited in the sense organs can give rise to sensations or real knowledge until they reach the brain.

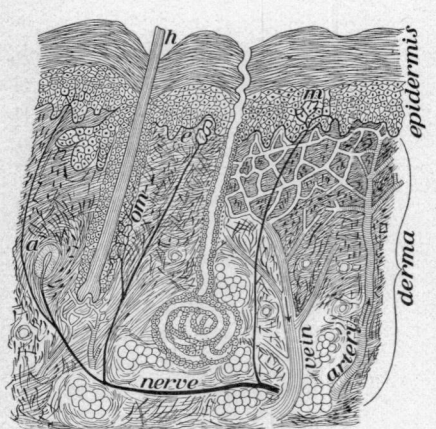

Fig. 124.—Thin slice through the skin to show nerve endings, *m, e* and *a*. Much enlarged.

The Kinds of Senses.—There are two general classes of senses. The *inner* or *general senses* are those telling a person of the condition of the body. To this class belong the senses of hunger, pain, thirst, and weariness. The *outer* or *special senses* are those receiving the news of heat, cold, pressure, smell, taste, hearing, and sight.

Senses of the Skin.—In all parts of the skin, there is one kind of end organ for *pain*, another for *pressure*, another for *heat* and still a different one for *cold* sensations. These organs are little bulbs or other simple structures, too small to be seen without a microscope. They are of great use as they tell us when the body is too hot or too cold or when it is being hurt. The end organs of pain are present in many other parts of the body besides the skin.

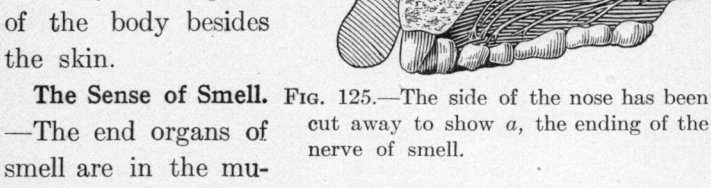

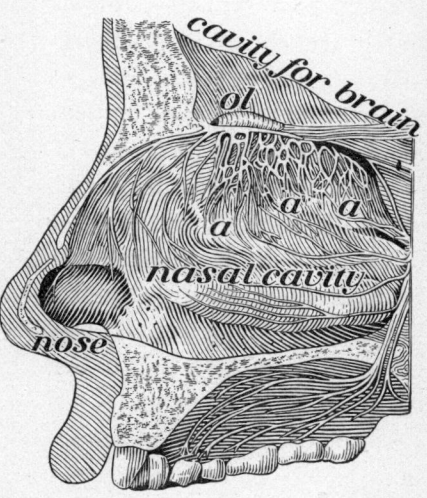

FIG. 125.—The side of the nose has been cut away to show *a*, the ending of the nerve of smell.

The Sense of Smell.—The end organs of smell are in the mucous membrane of the upper part of the cavity of the nose. They are affected only by substances which have odor. Their use is to help one to tell when food is fit to be eaten, when air is pure, and to give more pleasure in the eating of food with appetizing odors. In case of cold, mucus collects on the organs of smell and they are squeezed up by the swollen mucous membrane, so that they are of little use.

The Sense of Taste.—The sense organs of taste lie in the mucous membrane of the tongue and other regions of the mouth. They are tiny oval bodies called *taste buds* from which nerve fibers lead to the brain.

A substance can arouse the sense of taste only when in the form of a liquid or dissolved in a liquid. It is therefore important that all food should be chewed many times and dissolved as completely as possible in the mouth, so as to affect the sense of taste. This causes the gastric juice to flow abundantly.

The Sense of Hearing.—The organs of hearing are the ears. Each one consists of three parts, named the *outer ear*, the *middle ear* and the *inner ear*. The outer ear is composed of the *pinna* sticking out from the side of the head to catch the sound, and the tube an inch long, extending inward. Across the inner end of the tube is a thin membrane, named the *tympanic membrane*.

The *middle ear* or *tympanum* is called the *ear drum* because it is somewhat like a drum. It contains air which may pass in and out through the tube leading to the throat. The mouth of the tube is usually closed, but it opens every time a bit of food or even saliva is swallowed. Three bones form a chain stretching from the outer membrane, which is the tympanic membrane of the middle ear, to the inner membrane closing a small oval opening into the internal ear (Fig. 126).

ORGANS FOR RECEIVING KNOWLEDGE 177

The *inner ear* is deep in the temporal bone. It consists chiefly of three tubes forming half circles, a tube coiled like a snail shell, and a little cavity into which the four

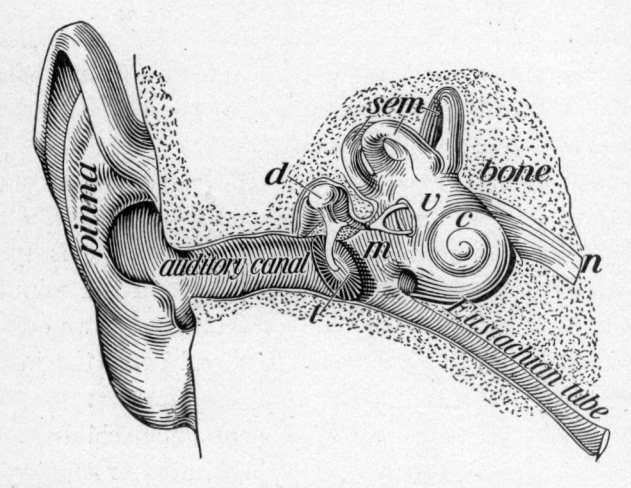

FIG. 126.—The ear. *m*, middle ear; *d*, bone of the middle ear; *t*, membrane of the ear drum; *n*, nerve of hearing; *sem* and *c*, canals forming the inner ear.

tubes open. These parts are filled with fluid and surrounded on the outside with a watery fluid.

How We Hear.—The tap of a bell or any other sound makes little waves in the air much like the waves made in water by casting in a pebble. These air waves strike on the outer membrane of the ear drum and make it move the chain of bones in the middle ear. The bones then move the inner membrane so that it makes waves in the fluid of the inner ear to strike on the organ of hearing. This feeling aroused by the waves is carried by the nerve of hearing to the brain which has learned to know the meaning of each kind of wave.

The Care of the Ears.—Hard objects, such as pencils and sticks, should not be pushed into the outer ear for fear of breaking the ear drum. The wax which tends to keep insects and dirt from lodging on the tympanum sometimes collects in too large quantities in the canal. It may then be removed with a soft moist cloth.

Insects finding their way into the canal of the outer ear may be killed or made to come out by putting in a few drops of warm soapy water while the patient is lying down with the affected ear uppermost. In ten minutes after the water is in, the ear should be turned down on the pillow when the water will flow out and carry the insect with it.

Ear Ache.—This is a common ailment among children. It is sometimes caused by sitting in the wind after running or playing. Sleeping so that the wind blows on the head may also produce ear ache. Another common cause is the presence of spongy growths called *adenoids* in the upper part of the throat at the back of the nose. They close the opening of the tube leading from the throat to the ear (Fig. 75). A physician should be consulted.

Deafness.—The ear is a very delicate organ, and injury to any of its parts may cause deafness. A sudden pull or a sharp slap on the ear may break the ear drum. In many cases nature will mend this break. Water should be kept out of the ears when diving, by inserting a wad of raw cotton or wool. Closure of the tube extending from the throat to the ear, by catarrh, sometimes causes partial deafness. A growth of germs in the tympanum producing an inflammation as in running ears, may make the three little bones grow together so that they cannot move freely to transmit sound.

More than half of the school children in the United States suffer from some ailment of the ears, eyes, nose or throat. This fact shows the great need of giving proper care to these delicate sense organs. After some diseases, such as scarlet fever, special attention must be given to the ears to avoid partial deafness.

Testing the Hearing.—Many children are partly deaf without knowing it. The hearing of every child should be tested occasionally, so that any deafness coming on may be discovered early, when it can be remedied. Each ear should be tested separately by holding a thickly folded handkerchief over the other one. For testing use the tick of a watch or a clock. Children who appear dull often have the best minds, but do not hear distinctly.

Curing Deafness.—The deaf and dumb are unable to hear because the ending of the sense organ in the inner ear is imperfect. Some cases of deafness resulting from disease or accident can be cured, but one should never pay attention to the numerous advertisements in newspapers and magazines offering to cure all sorts of deafness. They are the words of quack doctors who rob people of thousands of dollars and are likely to damage the ear seriously. An honest physician does not advertise a sure cure for deafness, but does all in his power to help his patients.

The Sense of Sight.—More knowledge is received through

the sense of sight than by all other senses combined. It is a wise provision that we should have two ears and two eyes, for if one is injured the other can do duty for both.

The end organs for sight are the two eyeballs connected behind with the pair of *optic nerves* leading to the brain.

The Eyeball.—The eyeballs are fixed in soft cushions of fat in the two cavities in the front of the skull. Each eyeball is a globe held in place by six muscles and the optic nerve. The muscles cause the movements of the eyeball.

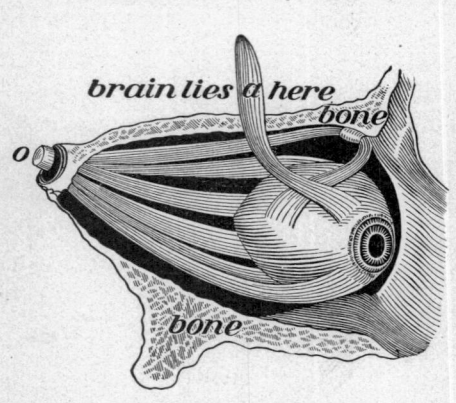

How the Eyeball is Protected.—The eyebrows on the lower part of the forehead prevent the sweat from running on to the eyeball, and the *eyelids* keep out dirt and too strong light, and other agents that might cause injury. The *eyelashes* on the edge of the lids are very sensitive so that the least touch on them causes the eye to be closed.

FIG. 127.—The eye with its muscles. The side of the skull is cut away. *o*, the nerve of sight.

The *tear gland* at the upper and outer corner of the eye makes a slightly salty fluid to keep the surface of the eyeball moist and to wash away dust. A tube, the tear duct, carries the tears from the inner corner of the eye into the nose.

ORGANS FOR RECEIVING KNOWLEDGE

Parts of the Eyeball.—The outer covering of the eyeball is a tough coat which is as transparent as glass in front. The transparent part is called the *cornea*. Just back of the cornea is a curtain, the *iris*, which has in it a round hole, the *pupil*, to admit light. The color of the iris gives the brown, black or blue color to the eye.

The outer coat of the eye except the cornea is lined with a thin black membrane, to keep the light from scattering about after it strikes the inner surface of the eyeball. Lying close against this black membrane is a tender pink membrane, known as the *retina*. This is the real organ upon which the rays of light make an impression to be carried to the brain.

Contents of the Eyeball.—The cavity of the eyeball is filled with three different substances

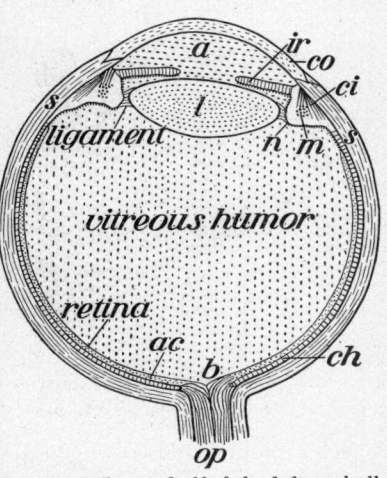

FIG. 128.—Lower half of the left eyeball. *a*, watery humor; *b*, entrance of the nerve of sight, *op*; *ci*, muscles to change the lens for near sight; *ir*, iris; *co*, cornea; *l*, lens; *ch*, black membrane.

called *humors*. They are as clear as glass. The middle one and the most firm of all is the *crystalline lens*, about twice as large and about the shape of a red cinnamon drop. It is held in place just back of the iris by means of a ligament fixed to the black membrane. The cavity in front of this lens is filled with a *watery humor* while the much larger cavity back of it is occupied by a clear jellylike mass. All these parts of the eyeball may be seen by getting from the butcher or slaughter house the eye of an ox or pig and cutting it open.

How We See.—In order to see an object clearly, the light from it must be brought to a focus on the retina. The *focus* is the point at which all rays of light meet as when one holds a burning glass over the hand and brings the rays of the sun together in one tiny spot on the hand. Any transparent substance with outward curving or convex surfaces will bring the rays of light to a focus. The crystalline lens, therefore, brings the rays of light to a focus on the retina. This gives an impression which the optic nerve can carry to the brain.

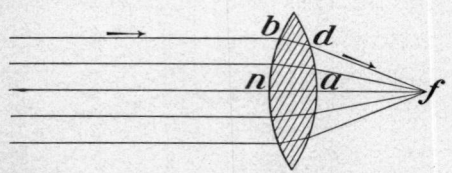

FIG. 129.—The rays of light passing through a convex lens *bd* are brought to a focus at *f*.

Why Some Persons Cannot See Clearly.—Very few grown persons have perfect sight, and many children cannot see distinctly objects unless they are held very near to the eye. Pupils who must hold this book nearer than 16 inches to the eye to read easily, without eye strain, are nearsighted. Those who must hold the book nearly two feet from the eyes when reading are farsighted.

Nearsightedness is usually due to the fact that the eye is too long from before backward. Farsightedness is caused by the eye being too short from before backward.

The Use of Glasses.—Many persons after reading or

studying an hour have headache, and tears gather in the eyes because they have been strained to see clearly. The muscle controlling the shape of the crystalline lens was worked hard to bring the rays of light to a focus on the retina. Such a difficulty can be remedied by wearing glasses.

When the glasses suit the eyes properly, one can read without headache or eye strain. *Nearsightedness* is remedied by using concave glasses, that is, glasses with both surfaces curving inward toward each other. *Farsightedness* is aided by convex glasses which have the surfaces curving outward.

How Children Injure Their Eyes.— Examination shows that at six years of age four fifths of the pupils have perfect sight, and only four out of a hundred have very bad eyes.

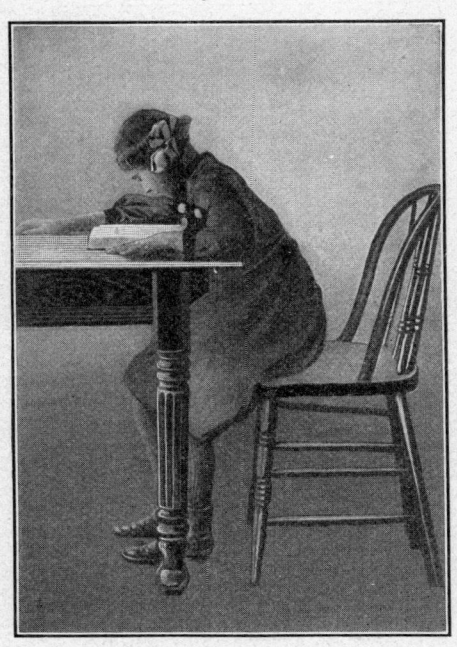

FIG. 130.—How the eyes are injured.

At eight years of age three fourths of the pupils have perfect eyes and eight out of a hundred have very imperfect eyes. At eleven years of age only about two thirds of the pupils have perfect eyes. This shows that most children begin life with good eyes, but hurt them by improper use.

Many children weaken their eyes by reading in a dim light, reading in bed, or with the head hanging over the book so that there is pressure on the sides of the eyeball. Studying books or maps with fine print is injurious to the eyes. Smoking much tobacco sometimes makes the eyes weak.

How to Keep the Eyes Strong.—The book should never be held nearer to the eyes than one foot, and the reading of print finer than that in this book should be avoided by young children. Keep the head erect when studying, and hold the book up. If the eyes ache or smart, stop using them for several hours. Never read in a dim light.

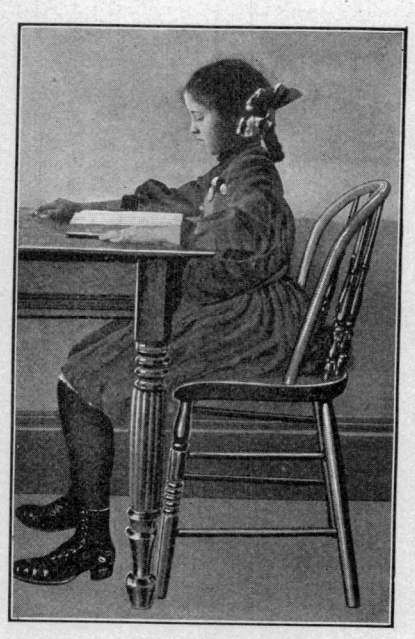

Fig. 131.—Proper position at the table to prevent eyestrain.

When recovering from measles, chicken pox and other diseases, the eyes should not be used in reading or sewing, and should be shielded from a strong light. In seeking help for weak eyes consult a reliable oculist, and give no heed to the large advertisements by eye specialists offering to furnish glasses cheap. Poor glasses may ruin the eyes.

Common Injuries to the Eye.—Cinders and other bits of dirt often get beneath the eyelid. Do not rub the eye. Holding the opposite eye shut and blowing the nose vigorously a few times, will often remove the dirt. By looking down, another person may seize the edge of the upper lid and turn it backward over a rounded match stick. The dirt can then be removed with the corner of a clean handkerchief. The lower lid may be merely drawn down to clean off the surface.

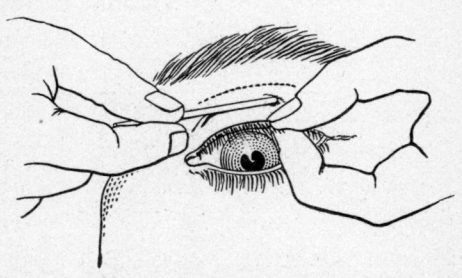

Fig. 132.—How a match stick may be used to turn up an injured lid for examination.

Sore Eyes.—When the eyes are red or inflamed from any cause, some relief may be had by bathing them several times daily with a solution of boracic acid. This is made by dissolving in a teacupful of water as much boracic acid as will lie on a silver half-dollar.

Sore eyes are usually much relieved by being washed out with the boracic acid solution, because this tends to keep from growing the germs which cause the trouble. Care should be taken that the germs in the sore eyes do not get on pencils, towels or handkerchiefs used by other persons, and thus make their eyes sick.

Cataract is a growth in the crystalline lens making it opaque. It can be cured only by an operation by a surgeon.

How Narcotics Affect the Sense Organs.—Much chewing and smoking tends to lessen the sense of taste. Smoking may also decrease the sense of smell by irritating the delicate end organs in the nose. Smoking prepares the way for catarrh in the young. This may affect not only the sense of smell, but also that of hearing, by extending up the tube leading to the middle ear.

Frequent smoking in the young has been known to affect the sight seriously. Doctor Alfred Woodhull of the United States Army, says: "Tobacco is liable to render vision weak and uncertain, causing objects to appear nebulous, or it creates the sensation of floating spots." One well known eye specialist alone reports 35 cases of injured vision produced by the continual irritation of the optic nerve by tobacco.

Doctor McSherry says when sight fails in smokers and no change in structure can be seen, tobacco poisoning may be assumed. Candidates for the United States Naval Academy, rejected on account of poor eyesight, have in most cases admitted using tobacco while young.

The period of life before twenty is the time when the sense organs are most markedly affected by the use of tobacco and alcoholic drinks. Even later in life narcotics may do lasting injury to the senses. The use of much liquor produces bloodshot eyes, because the walls of the arteries are relaxed, and so become enlarged.

Long use of intoxicants has been known to do permanent

injury to the optic nerve. This was probably due to the paralyzing effect of the alcohol on the nerves controlling the blood vessels leading to the eye.

Practical Questions

1. What are the sense organs? 2. Explain how we get acquainted with the nature of an apple. 3. Name eight senses. 4. Name three sense organs in the skin. 5. Of what use is the sense of smell? 6. Describe the sense of taste. 7. Name the three parts of the ear. 8. Describe the outer ear. 9. State three facts about the middle ear. 10. Describe the inner ear. 11. Explain how we hear. 12. How may insects be removed from the outer ear? 13. What causes ear ache? 14. What may cause deafness? 15. Can you hear a watch tick six feet distant with either ear closed? 16. What nerves lead from the eye to the brain? 17. Describe the tear gland. 18. Name the parts of the eyeball. 19. Give the contents of the eyeball. 20. Explain how light is brought to a focus. 21. What causes near sight and far sight? 22. How do glasses help one see? 23. Describe how children often injure their eyes. 24. Explain how to keep the eyes strong. 25. What care should be given sore eyes? 26. How does tobacco affect the sense organs?

CHAPTER XIX

THE CAUSE OF SICKNESS

The Work of Parasites.—Only one in every forty persons dies of old age. About twice that number meet death by accidents, while disease is responsible for over nine tenths of the deaths of the human race. The numerous diseases affecting man may be divided into two classes, known as *germ diseases* and *cell diseases*.

The germ diseases are caused by tiny plants or animals, called *parasites*, feeding upon the human body, which is their *host*. These parasites, the smaller of which are commonly called microbes or bacteria, make one ill chiefly by means of the poisonous matter which they give out. In Europe and America, 50,000,000 people are annually laid prostrate by germ diseases, which result in over 3,000,000 deaths.

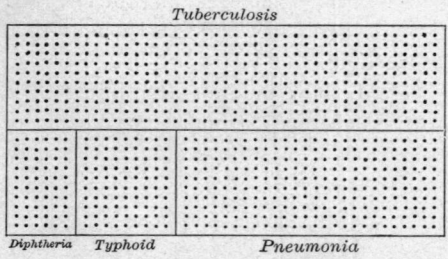

Fig. 133.—The black dots stand for the graves made daily in the United States for the people dying from the above diseases.

Kinds of Diseases.—Such ailments as consumption, smallpox, and scarlet fever, which may be contracted by breathing in the germs floating in the air, are called catching or *contagious diseases,* because the healthy acquire the disease by coming near where the sick are, or have been.

Sicknesses like yellow fever, lockjaw and malaria are not *contagious diseases,* for the reason that persons living in the same house and even sleeping in the same bed, with the sick do not become ill, unless a mosquito or a sharp instrument carries the germs from the sick to the well.

The cell diseases, such as alcoholism, diabetes, insanity, and cancer, are due to changed methods of work and growth on the part of the cells in certain regions of the body. More people die from germ diseases than from any other diseases. This means that most sickness results from tiny plants and animals growing within our bodies.

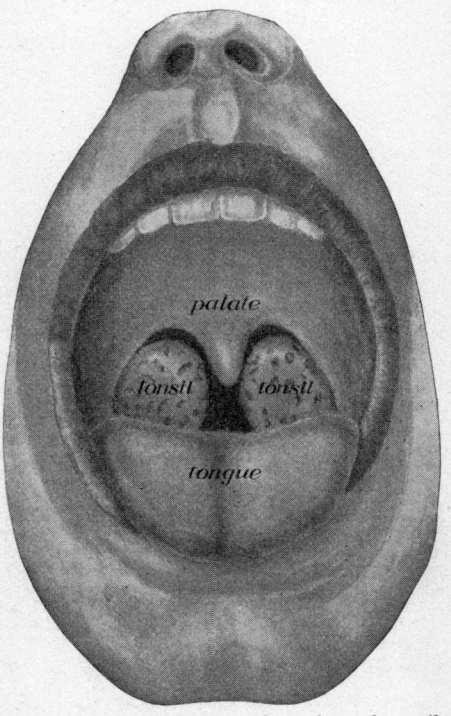

FIG. 134.—Drawing of the enlarged tonsils in a ten-year old boy. Disease germs may enter the system easily through such large soft tonsils. Thousands of germs of tuberculosis were found in the left tonsil.

The Discovery of What Causes Disease.—Several hundred

years ago disease was thought to be due to evil spirits, which took up their abode in the body. Here they produced continuous suffering, until driven out by various devices such as beating the patient with a strap, making hideous noises, or giving him medicine consisting of powdered bones and dried snakes.

Although for fifty years it has been thought by some that many diseases were due to bacteria, yet the fact that each of certain diseases is caused by a particular kind of bacteria was not clearly proved until 1876. In that year, Louis Pasteur, of France, showed that anthrax, a sickness of cattle, was caused by a rodlike plant. He got a few of these plants from the blood of a sick cow, planted them in broth, where they increased rapidly in number. A few were then injected under the skin of a healthy cow, which soon after became sick. In her blood the same plants were found in vast numbers. They were also found in all other sick cows examined, but never in well ones. These studies showed that this special kind of germ is always the cause of anthrax. In a similar manner, or by some other equally reliable method, it has been shown that each of the following ailments is produced by its own particular kind of germ: diphtheria, typhoid fever, malaria, pneumonia, leprosy, lockjaw, hydrophobia, grippe, erysipelas and tuberculosis.

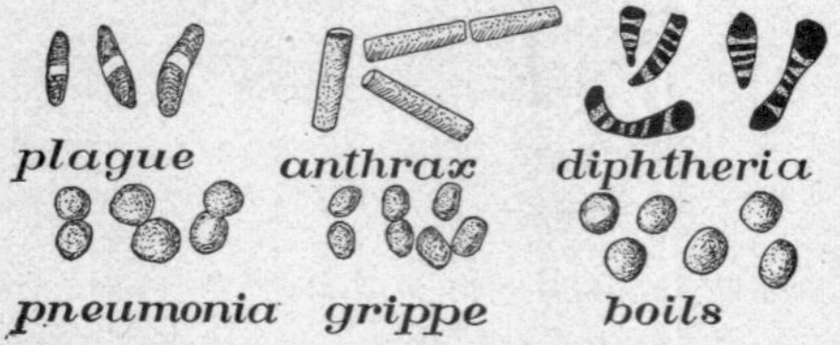

FIG. 135.—The bacteria of various diseases. Much enlarged.

plague *anthrax* *diphtheria*
pneumonia *grippe* *boils*

There is no doubt that measles, scarlet fever, smallpox and mumps are also produced by germs, but no one has yet been able to find them. Since all germ diseases may be prevented by keeping the germs out of the body, much effort has been made to learn how they gain entrance.

How Germs Enter the Body.—Safety from bad men, who rob and murder, depends largely upon keeping them out of our houses. The same is true of the germs that maim and kill. When we learn how they enter the body and then find a way to shut them out, they cannot harm us.

The germs of any contagious disease may be taken in by breathing, but other ways of entering the body are also known. Grippe, pneumonia, sore throat, and whooping cough are, no doubt, often caught by drinking from the same cup lately used by those just recovering from these diseases. Numerous disease germs as well as harmless ones may be present in the mouths of such patients. By examining, with a microscope, a glass touched by the lips as many as 20,000 bacteria have been found on it. More than five thousand germs have been found on a glass slip touched with the finger moistened with saliva, as when one does this to help turn the pages of a book. The fingers touching soiled books, clothing, pencils, or other things handled by the sick, may afterward serve to convey the germs to the mouth of the healthy.

How the Germs of Tuberculosis Enter the Body.—Tuberculosis commonly called consumption, frequently affects both cattle and man. Until 1905 it was thought to be generally acquired by breathing the germs into the lungs with the air. It has been lately shown, however, that the germs more often reach the lungs by passing through the walls of the alimentary canal into the lymph vessels and thence by the blood to the lungs. Here the thin-walled capillaries permit the germs to pass through into

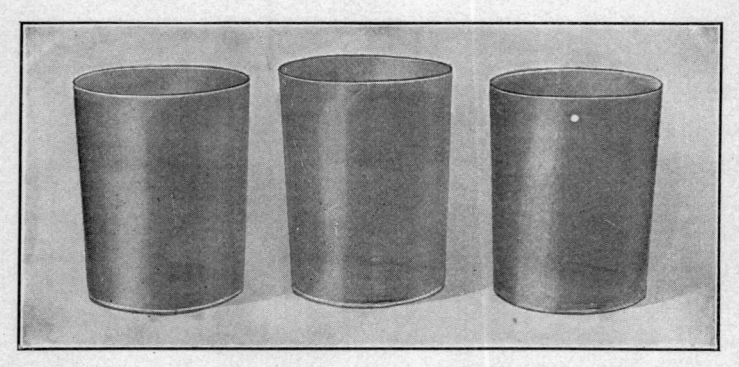

Fig. 136.—A clean glass and two glasses which had been used by many pupils. The microscope showed that the dirt on the two outer glasses consisted of saliva, dead bits of skin and millions of germs. From a photograph.

the tissues. The germs once in the body may lie there for twenty years without growing, or they may develop immediately.

Experiments Showing how Tuberculosis may be Caught.—The lungs of ten healthy guinea pigs fed on milk containing tubercle bacilli became in about two months, badly affected with tuberculosis. The tubercular germs injected under the skin of hogs and cows, in most cases, produced disease in the lungs. Calves fed on the milk of tuberculous cows, only a few days, acquired tuberculosis of the lungs.

The sputum or spit of tuberculous patients contains

millions of the disease germs. These may get on the furniture or drinking cup, or may be carried by flies from the spittoon to food, or may dry and be blown about in the wind. In any case they are liable to reach the mouth of a healthy person.

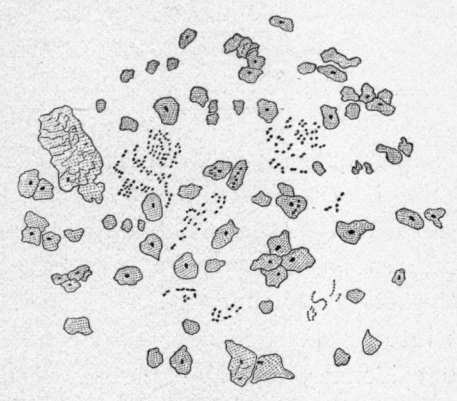

The Danger from Tuberculosis in Cows.—A large number of cows have tuberculosis, but it is not often detected by a farmer until the animals become very sick. Nearly one third of the cattle of Great Britain are said to have this disease, but it is much less common among the cows of the United States. Fortunately less than half of the sick animals shed the germs in their milk, but vast numbers of the deadly germs are found in their manure. Where

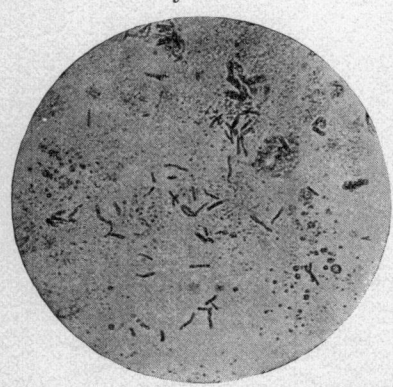

FIG. 137.—Drawing of a tiny circle on the glass at the right in Figure 136 as seen under the microscope. The larger bodies are bits of skin from the mouths of pupils who drank from the glass, and the little dots are germs from their mouths.

FIG. 138.—Germs of tuberculosis. Much enlarged. From a photograph.

the dairyman is careless this often soils the cow, then becomes dry, and is later brushed off into the milk pail.

Germs of tuberculosis have been frequently found in milk, and numerous cases are on record, where the use of milk from sick cows has given the disease to children.

Tubercular germs lodging in the lungs produce *consumption*; in the lymph glands, *scrofula*; in the skin, *lupus*; in the bones, *white swelling*, *hipjoint disease* or other trouble; and in the membranes of the brain and spinal cord, *meningitis*.

Typhoid Fever and Water.—The germs of typhoid fever get into the body in most cases with food or water. In 200 epidemics, during each of which from ten to one thousand three hundred people suffered with the fever, about three fourths were caused by water and the remainder by milk.

In the winter of 1885, the excreta from a single typhoid patient were cast out on the snow along the mountain stream supplying Plymouth, Pennsylvania, with water. During the first thaw of spring, the germs were carried with the melted snow into the reservoir. Two weeks later numerous cases of fever appeared daily in the town, until 1,104 persons were sick. More

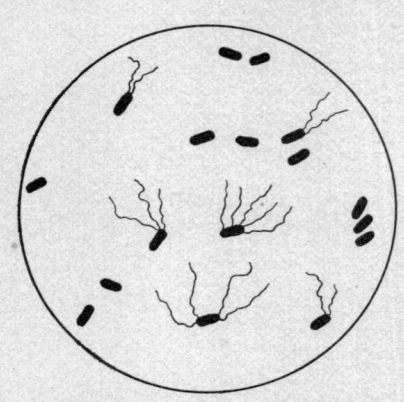

FIG. 139.—The germs causing typhoid fever. Much enlarged.

than one hundred of them died. This shows how wrong it is to allow the waste from the body to run into a stream likely to be used for drinking.

The scattered cases of typhoid occurring in many communities, may be due to a very slight pollution of the water, or to flies carrying the germs from sewers and other places to food.

Typhoid Fever Transmitted by Milk.—Many severe epidemics of fever have resulted from bad milk. As the cows never have this disease the germs must get into the milk from an outside source. This is often the water used from a shallow well or stream to wash the cans. A single germ clinging to the can is able to grow so rapidly as to produce a million germs within twelve hours.

Frequently germs have been known to get into the milk from the hands or clothes of those who have just recovered from the disease, or from those who have been nursing a typhoid patient.

Germ Diseases which are not Catching.—The germs of lockjaw are present in the soil, and other places, but can do no harm unless they get into a wound with the air shut out. *Boils* or any other inflammation are the result of bacteria gaining entrance and growing

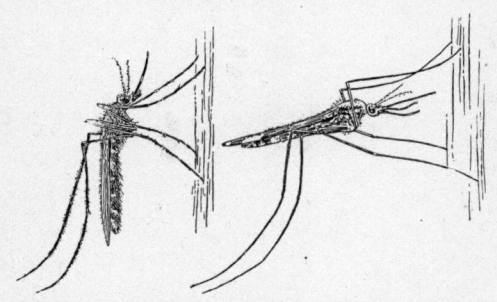

FIG. 140.—The common mosquito on the left and the malaria mosquito at the right. Note the difference in positions.

beneath the skin. Several diseases, including *hydrophobia, malaria, yellow fever* and *sleeping sickness,* are produced by tiny animals put into the blood by the bite of other larger animals.

Hydrophobia usually results from the bite of a rabid dog or cat, with the germs in their saliva. The parasites of malaria and yellow fever enter the body only by the bite of certain mosquitoes. The malaria mosquito may always be recognized by its spotted wings and the oblique position of its body to the upright support on which it alights. The germs of sleeping sickness are inserted by the bite of an African fly.

Cholera infantum and other sickness of the bowels in babies often result from the use of unclean milk and water.

Alcohol and Disease.—The habitual use of liquor weakens the cells of the body which naturally kill off the harmful germs. Recent studies clearly show that those using alcoholic drinks, except in very small quantities, are not only

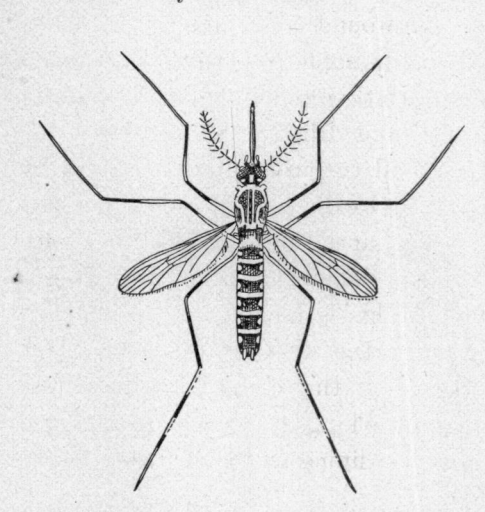

Fig. 141.—The mosquito which sucks the germs of yellow fever from the sick and then in biting healthy persons plants the germs in their blood.

attacked sooner than others with germ diseases, but are also less able to resist the effects of the disease.

The greatest Russian scientist has lately shown that alcohol paralyzes those elements in the body tending to prevent disease. By experimenting he found that in exposing rabbits to certain disease germs, only those animals which had been given alcohol ever contracted the disease.

Serious diseases of the liver, kidneys, blood vessels and heart often result from the long-continued use of beer or whisky.

Alcohol and Wounds.—Persons hurt by serious cuts or bruises do not usually die because of loss of blood, but because germs enter the wound and poison the body. Injuries to persons daily drinking beer or whisky are much more likely to result in death than the same kind of injuries to those abstaining from strong drink. This is because the guard cells, the white blood corpuscles, which collect by millions in a wound, are hurt by the alcohol and cannot perform their duty any better than a drunken soldier on guard.

Alcohol and Pneumonia.—Pneumonia is a deadly disease among drinking people. This is largely due to the fact that alcohol has weakened the white blood cells, which tend to destroy the germs of this disease. Alcohol also causes the blood vessels of the lungs to become more gorged with blood, and the mucous lining of the air tubes to become more inflamed.

Alcohol and Cholera.—In the Old World cholera kills thousands every month in the year. Those who have studied the disease, say that strong drink is an important factor in weakening the body, so that the germs may begin their deadly work.

In a cholera epidemic in England, the death rate was four times as great among the drinkers attacked as among those abstaining from alcoholic beverages, such as beer and whisky.

Alcohol and Tuberculosis.—This disease causes 5,000,000 deaths yearly in the world. Scientists, who have been studying the cause for this great sacrifice, declare that if the use of alcoholic drinks were stopped the number of deaths from tuberculosis would soon decrease one half.

In a large hospital for consumptives it was found that only six in every hundred persons had been living without the use of alcoholic drink. In a certain district in France where much wine is used, ten out of every thousand inhabitants die yearly of tuberculosis. In other districts where very little wine is used, only three persons out of each thousand living, die of this disease.

How Alcohol Causes Tuberculosis.—Liquor always weakens the body cells, which in health are strong enough to eat the tubercle germs. Persons who spend money for drink are often unable to get a sufficient supply of good food. Lack of food makes the body weak, and, therefore, an easy prey to the disease. The natural appetite for food is sometimes deadened by alcoholic drink, so that too little real nourishment is taken to make the body strong.

Practical Questions

1. What causes most deaths? 2. What is a contagious disease?
3. Name some contagious diseases. 4. Who proved that certain

germs cause disease? 5. Explain how it was proved that a certain germ causes anthrax. 6. Name eight diseases caused by germs. 7. How may all germ diseases be prevented? 8. Name five ways in which germs may get into the body. 9. Explain how germs of tuberculosis enter the body. 10. Describe an experiment showing how tuberculosis may be caught. 11. Why is there danger from tuberculosis in cows? 12. Name several diseases caused by tubercular germs. 13. How do the germs of typhoid fever usually enter the body? 14. Tell how the germs from one person caused the fever in over 1,000 others. 15. How do the fever germs get into milk? 16. Name some germ diseases which are not catching. 17. How do the germs of malaria and yellow fever enter the body? 18. What causes cholera infantum? 19. How may alcohol cause disease? 20. Why does alcohol make pneumonia worse? 21. What fact shows that alcohol makes cholera more severe? 22. Show that alcohol is a cause of tuberculosis.

Suggestions for the Teacher

By addressing the State Board of Health at the Capital of the state, numerous pamphlets on the prevention of disease may be secured free of charge. The following circulars on health may be had free by requesting them from the United States Department of Agriculture: Tubercle Bacilli in Butter; How Insects Affect Health in Rural Districts; Bacteria in Milk; Sanitary Milk Production; Facts about Milk. Many of the popular magazines also have timely articles relating to the cause and prevention of disease. From these several sources the children may gather many valuable facts which can be made the basis of short essays or language exercises and read before the class.

CHAPTER XX

HOW TO KEEP WELL

Healthy Living.—Eating the proper kind of food, and chewing it thoroughly, taking plenty of exercise, and breathing deeply fresh air, are great aids in keeping the body strong and well. Good habits and cheerfulness invite health and happiness. Unless care is used, however, some of the germs of disease are likely to get into the body, and then they may grow and cause sickness.

Fighting our Enemies.—In pioneer days, the foe of life was Indians and wild beasts. To-day it is the countless unseen life that makes human flesh its prey. Safety lies only in making ourselves the conquerors.

There are three kinds of warfare used in fighting germ diseases. One kind is to destroy the harmful germs in the excretions leaving the body. A second plan is to stop the disease germs scattered about by careless people, from entering the body. A third means of keeping away disease is to develop substances in the body able to kill the unfriendly germs entering.

Destroying the Cause of Disease.—Until 1890 but little attention was given to the several means of preventing sickness. A sure method of restraining criminals from robbing and killing, is to keep them shut up in prisons, or kill them. Likewise a certain method of preventing deadly germs from robbing some citizens of health and killing others, is to destroy the germs when they leave the body of the sick.

It is in the spit, and the bowel and kidney excretions that the harmful germs generally escape from a patient. For this reason all waste matter from the sick should be so treated as to kill the germs in it. This may be done by adding to it an equal amount of 5% formalin or a large quantity of boiling water. Any germ killer is called a *disinfectant*. The killing of germs is *disinfecting*. Carbolic acid, sunshine, and cresol are disinfectants. The time required for the disinfectant to kill the germs is about two hours.

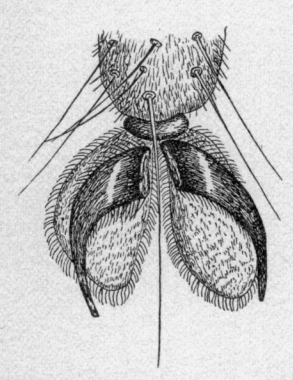

FIG. 142.—The foot of a fly showing the hairs to which thousands of germs cling to be carried to food over which the insect walks. Much enlarged.

How Carelessness Destroys Health.—Nearly three hundred thousand cases of typhoid fever occur annually in this country, resulting in about forty thousand deaths. Three fourths of this suffering and loss of life is due to negligence in permitting the living typhoid germs in the excretions of the sick to escape into the streams, wells and soil. Flies are known to carry on their feet and scatter over food the disease germs allowed to escape from the bodies of patients.

When, a few years ago, less than a thousand human beings, on a vessel near New York, lost their lives through the carelessness of others, the whole country was aroused and demanded that those who neglected their duty should be punished. Every year more than one hundred thousand men, women and children lose their lives, because others neglect their duty to kill the deadly germs passing from the bodies of those sick with contagious diseases.

The farmer can get no wheat unless he sows the seed, and it is equally true that there can be no germ diseases unless the germs are sown by the sick. It should be remembered that the disease germs often continue in the waste given off by the sick for a month or more after recovery. This is especially true of diphtheria and typhoid fever.

Caring for the Sick.—A person suffering from a contagious disease should not mingle with well persons. He should be placed in a large airy room shut off from the rest of the house as much as possible and exposed to the sun, which is the best of germ killers. The hangings and carpets and all unnecessary furniture should be removed. Only the nurse and doctor are to be allowed to enter the room. No clothing, dishes, or other articles should be taken from the room without being soaked in boiling water, or other germ killer like 5% formalin.

Care of the Sick Room.—After touching a patient, or handling his clothing, the hands should be thoroughly washed with hot water and soap. The clothing and dishes used about the sick must be boiled. Toys handled by a scarlet fever patient have been known to give the disease to others more than a year later. The room should not be swept, but wiped up daily with a cloth wrung out in a quart of water to which a half-pint of 5% formalin has been added. Screens should be used to prevent the entrance of flies which may distribute the disease germs.

When the patient has recovered, his entire body, including the hair, should be well washed with hot water and soap. As soon as the patient has left the room, it should be disinfected by the health officer, or some other person who understands the use of formalin.

Aid from the Board of Health.—In every city and community there are several persons appointed by law to act as a *board of health*. It is their duty to help the people to keep well. One of their number is chosen as *health officer*. He should be notified by a family, or their physician, when any contagious disease occurs in their house. He will then, free of charge, help them to keep the disease from spreading and disinfect the house when the patient has recovered. All directions given by the health officer should be carefully obeyed.

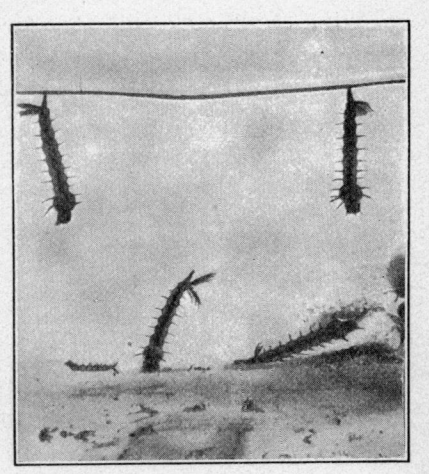

FIG. 143.—The young of mosquitoes called wigglers, living in stagnant water. From a photograph.

Keeping the Germs out of the Body.—With great care it is possible to keep out of the body the agents causing at least five of the germ diseases. The bacteria responsible for dysentery, cholera infantum and typhoid fever, may generally be avoided by keeping flies away from the food, and by drinking from clean vessels water or milk known to be pure, or by heating these fluids up to the boiling point. It is better to pasteurize questionable milk.

The use of boiled drinking water in Philadelphia, Cincinnati, Cleveland, Louisville, Memphis, New Orleans, St. Louis and Washington during the years 1900–1904 would have prevented 50,000 cases of typhoid fever. The use of boiled water in Pittsburg during the same five years would have prevented 10,000 cases of fever in that city.

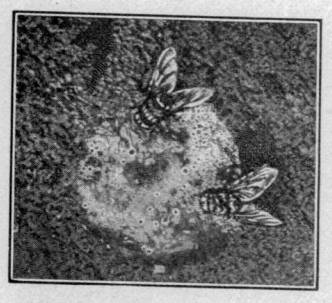

Fig. 144.—Flies at a feast. The germs in this spit will be carried by the insects to milk and other food which they seek later.

The germs of malaria and yellow fever are easily kept out of the system by preventing the two kinds of mosquitoes carrying them from biting. As the young of these insects live only in quiet pools of water, with no fish, their numbers may be much lessened by draining the puddles and pouring out the water in tubs and old cans. Where this cannot be done, the young may be killed by kerosene poured on the water, using one pint for every hundred square feet of surface (Fig. 143).

The terrible bubonic plague or black death, is conveyed to man by the bite of a flea or bug, living on rats and man.

Leprosy may also be caught by the bite of bed bugs or fleas.

Why Some Germs Cannot be Kept Out of the Body.—When near patients with scarlet fever, smallpox, grippe, measles, mumps and chicken pox, there is no way of shutting the germs out of the system, because they become mingled with the air. The germs of diphtheria and tuberculosis are also likely to mingle with the air, unless the patients use great care. The secretions of the mouth and nose should always be received into a cloth, or special pasteboard cup, and burned, and a cloth, to be later burned, should be held over the mouth while coughing. In quiet breathing no germs of any kind are given off.

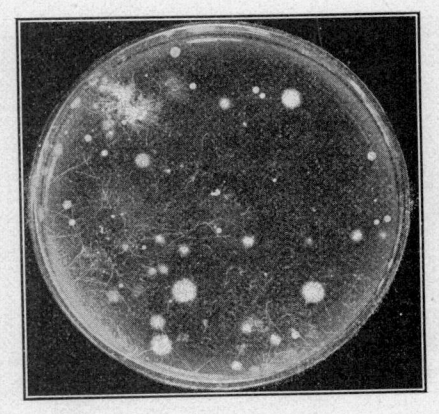

FIG. 145.—A dish of pure meat jelly over which a fly walked. Each white spot shows where a germ was scraped off its feet and grew two days later into millions.

How Germs are Removed from Water.—Many cities getting their water from streams likely to contain disease germs, pass the water through a layer of sand and coarse gravel. This is called a *filter*. The passing of water through it is *filtration*. The filter keeps back over nine tenths of the germs and they soon die. The small house filters are also useful, but they should be cleaned daily and boiled weekly.

Since the city sand filter has been in use at Albany, New York, only one fourth as many deaths occur yearly from typhoid fever as previously, and there have been less than half as many deaths from diarrheal diseases as formerly. At Lawrence, Massachusetts, only one fourth as many cases of typhoid fever occur yearly as before the water was filtered.

How the Body Tissues Kill Germs.—There is no doubt that disease germs get into the mouth and nose every day. The bacteria causing sore throat and pneumonia have been frequently found in the mouth and throat of healthy people. These germs are most likely to bring on disease, only when one becomes chilled, so that the body cells are weakened and permit the intruders to get a start.

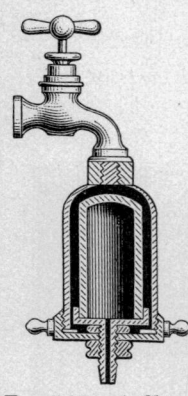

FIG. 146.—A filter to strain out the germs at the house tap. Such a filter must be cleaned and boiled weekly.

In health, the nasal mucus, gastric juice and blood are able to destroy vast numbers of bacteria. Certain other agents in the blood weaken bacteria gaining entrance, so that they are easily devoured by the white blood corpuscles.

Alcohol is the Foe of Health.—The following paragraphs are copied from large cards hung by the government authorities of Paris, in public waiting rooms, in order to check the waste of health caused by drinking wine, brandy and other liquors: "Alcoholism is chronic poisoning resulting from the habitual use of alcohol, even when this is not taken in amounts sufficient to produce drunkenness."

"The habit of drinking leads to the neglect of family, to forgetfulness of all social duties, to distaste for work, to want, theft, and crime. It leads, at the very least, to the hospital—for alcoholism causes a great variety of diseases, many of them most deadly: paralysis, insanity, disorders of the stomach and liver, dropsy; it is one of the frequent causes of consumption. Finally it complicates and renders more serious every acute illness; as typhoid fever, pneumonia, or erysipelas, which would be mild in a sober individual, will rapidly kill the alcoholic."

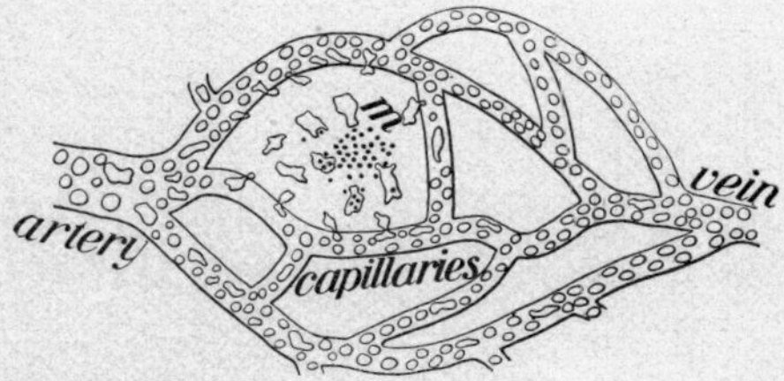

FIG. 147.—White blood corpuscles creeping out of the capillaries to eat the germs m about to cause a boil.

How the Body Becomes Safe from Some Diseases.—Safety from some diseases depends upon the germ-killing power of the blood. This power against some germs, such as those of tuberculosis, may be developed by using good food, taking plenty of sleep, an abundance of fresh air and regular exercise. The germ-killing power of the blood against the germs of such diseases as diphtheria, smallpox, lockjaw and hydrophobia may be developed by the use of antitoxin or by vaccination.

Tuberculosis.—The tiny plants causing this sickness are so abundant everywhere that it is impossible for those living in towns and cities to keep them out of the body. More than half of the people over 25 years of age have, at some time, had growing in their tissues the parasites causing tuberculosis. The fact that 400 people are dying daily in the United States, from this disease, and that one third of all deaths occurring between the ages of 15 and 45 years result from tuberculosis, shows the need of trying to render the body safe from disease.

How to Avoid Tuberculosis.—The right kind of living

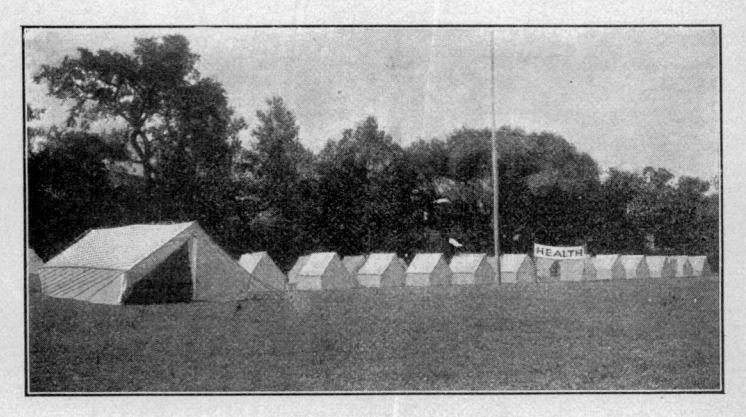

FIG. 148.—One way of strengthening the germ-killing power of the blood to fight off tuberculosis.

will, in nearly all persons, make the body able to kill any germs of tuberculosis that enter. The living and working rooms must be well ventilated. A window in the bedroom should be opened a foot both at the top and bottom in winter, and twice as much when the weather is not cold. Good food, including plenty of milk and eggs should be taken. Exercise, especially such as calls into action the chest muscles and fills the lungs with air, ought to be indulged in a half hour or more daily, with additional walks or games in the open air. Twelve-year old children should not have less than nine hours of sound sleep daily. Those who follow these rules of life will not suffer from tuberculosis. Three fourths of the half million persons with the disease in this country have been overworked, underfed, or lived in poorly ventilated rooms, with the sunshine shut out.

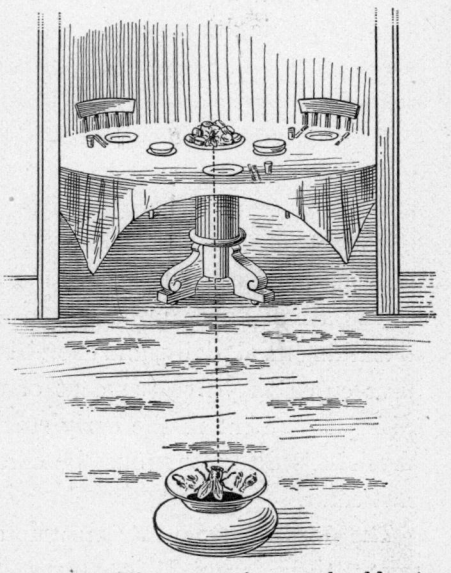

FIG. 149.—Why open spittoons should not be used by a consumptive, or anyone else.

How to Cure Tuberculosis. — A pain in the chest, a hacking cough, especially in the morning, rusty or blood-streaked sputum, loss in weight, and weariness and feverishness in the afternoon, are strong evidences of tuberculosis if they continue several weeks. A physician should be consulted.

Long experience has shown that no patent medicine or other preparation advertised in the papers with the exception of codliver-oil compounds, is of any use whatever for the consumptive. Some may seem to help for a time, because of the alcohol or other tonic they contain, but the help is only temporary. Many of them hasten the progress of the disease. The use of beer or whisky or any other alcoholic drink advertised to cure consumption, only makes it worse, because the alcohol has been shown to weaken the germ-killing power of the blood.

The one treatment which has been tried by over one hundred thousand patients and found most successful, is living a hygienic life to increase the germ-killing power of the blood. Keeping in the fresh air day and night, drinking daily a half gallon or more of rich milk and swallowing a half dozen raw eggs, in addition to eating three nourishing meals daily, and exercising according to strength, have cured fifty-five per cent of the tubercular patients taking treatment in the early stages of the disease. The physician's directions must be carefully followed in every particular.

The Danger from a Consumptive.—If proper care is taken, there is but little danger of catching consumption from living in the same house with a patient. No germs are given off in ordinary breathing. In coughing, a cloth to be later burned, should be held before the mouth. The sputum must be received into a shaving mug half filled with lye and scalded out daily, or into a paraffined paper cup with a cover to keep out the flies. The cup should be burned at the end of the day. More than ten million germs are known to be given off daily by some patients. The eating and drinking utensils must be placed in boiling water immediately after being used by the patient.

Where it is possible, a consumptive should go to a *sanatorium* or *hospital*. These are homes with doctors and nurses who thoroughly understand how to treat the sick to get the best results. Some of these homes receive poor persons free of charge.

Vaccination for Smallpox.—Before the year 1798, when Jenner showed the use of vaccination, smallpox was the worst of human ills. Scarcely any one lived beyond the age of thirty years without being attacked by the disease. One in every seven who suffered from it died, while many others were made deaf or blind.

In 1721 more than half of the inhabitants of Boston had smallpox, and a few years later 18,000 of the 50,000 residents of Greenland died of the malady. It killed 60,000,000 inhabitants of Europe in the eighteenth century.

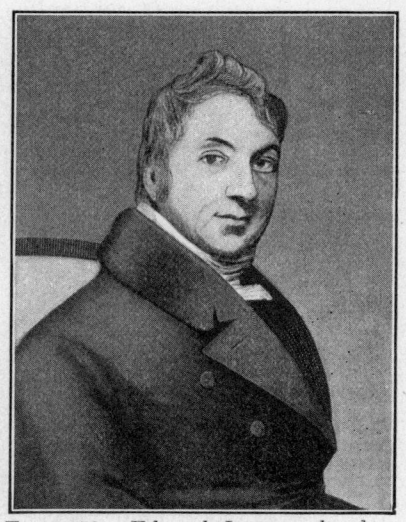

FIG. 150.—Edward Jenner who has saved thousands of lives by showing us how to prevent smallpox.

To-day smallpox is a rare disease, because vaccination properly performed absolutely prevents it. In Germany, where the law compels every person to be vaccinated twice, the deaths from smallpox are only one twentieth as great in proportion to the population, as they are in the

United States. Hundreds of people die yearly in our country from smallpox, because they neglect vaccination. Everyone, unless in ill health, should be vaccinated in infancy and again ten or twelve years later or oftener, if near a case of smallpox.

There is no danger of giving to one any disease by vaccination when the process is properly done, as the vaccine is now taken from healthy calves. If a clean instrument is used on a clean arm, with clean clothing, much of the soreness and inflammation may be avoided.

Antitoxin.—Other means of preventing some diseases or curing them are by using antitoxins, secured from the blood of domestic animals, treated in a special way. A puncture of the flesh by a dirty nail, or the common Fourth of July accidents in which powder is blown beneath the skin should receive the attention of a physician, who may use antitoxin to prevent lockjaw.

Diptheria antitoxin used in the early stages of the disease of diphtheria is a sure cure in nearly all cases. It saves yearly the lives of 45,000 children in Germany, and the lives of more than ten thousand persons in the United States.

If all persons obeyed strictly the teachings of this book for healthful living, there would be much less need of antitoxins and other drugs. Instead of the 5,000,000 homes now saddened yearly by sickness, the number might be decreased one half. It is better to prevent sickness than to try to cure it after it has come through our own carelessness.

Every boy and girl can be a life saver, and show true

patriotism by having the courage to live a healthful life and help others to do the same.

Practical Questions

1. What helps us keep well? 2. What are the three ways of fighting the germ diseases? 3. Name a sure way of preventing your germs from harming others. 4. What is a disinfectant? 5. Name two disinfectants. 6. What causes so much typhoid fever? 7. How could we get rid of all germ diseases? 8. Describe caring for the sick. 9. Why should you wash your hands after touching a sick person or his clothing? 10. How should clothing and dishes used about the sick be treated? 11. What is the duty of the board of health? 12. Give five ways of keeping the germs out of the body. 13. Why should all ponds containing mosquitoes be drained? 14. Why are fleas and bugs to be feared? 15. Why is it difficult to keep some germs out of the body? 16. What is filtration? 17. Show how filtering water saves lives. 18. Why do many germs entering the body cause no harm sometimes? 19. Explain how alcohol is the foe of health. 20. How may the body become safe from some diseases? 21. Tell how tuberculosis may be avoided. 22. What helps cure tuberculosis? 23. How may the danger from a consumptive be avoided? 24. What was the result of smallpox before the time of vaccination? 25. Why is there less smallpox in Germany than in our country? 26. Name two diseases in which antitoxin is used. 27. How many lives saved yearly in Germany by the use of antitoxin? 28. How many times have you been sick in your life? 29. How would the knowledge in this book have helped you prevent any of your sickness?

Suggestions for the Teacher

In connection with this chapter, the teacher may direct some valuable lessons in nature study. The life history of fleas, mosquitoes and flies should be studied. All information needed may be found in pamphlets issued free by the United States Department of Agriculture or secured from any recent elementary textbook on zoölogy. It is important that every one should have a practical knowledge of these three kinds of insects which are responsible for transmitting diseases afflicting more than 1,000,000 persons annually in the United States and its possessions.

From May until November, the eggs and the two young stages of the mosquito may be found in pools of water or even in pails or tubs left standing a week or two out of doors. In malaria and yellow fever districts, special attention should be given to the means of destroying the young mosquitoes. The children may be asked to report in how many places they find mosquitoes breeding. Some communities have spent thousands of dollars yearly in cleaning out the breeding places of mosquitoes.

The boys may be asked to find out where the young of flies called maggots live in their neighborhood. These pests may be found in horse manure, uncovered garbage cans and other kinds of decaying matter. Let the pupils suggest means of getting rid of flies when they have learned that they can breed only in waste matter.

The care of the teeth, the chewing of food and the use of cold baths and fresh air in making strong bodies should be emphasized. A health talk by a physician to the entire school is always helpful and a great aid in impressing upon the pupils the value of a sound body.

PRONUNCIATION AND EXPLANATION

OF

DIFFICULT WORDS

Ad'e noids: spongy growths at the back part of the nose.

Al bu'min: the largest part of the solid matter in lean meat and white of egg.

Al'co hol: a substance formed by yeast growing in a sweet solution.

Al'co hol ism: a disease caused by using much strong drink.

A nat'o my: the study treating of the parts of the body.

An ti tox'in: a substance which prevents certain poisons given off by bacteria from harming the body.

A or'ta: the chief artery in the trunk. It is in front of the backbone.

Ap'o plex y: sudden loss of motion and fainting caused by the clogging or bursting of a blood vessel in the brain.

A sy'lum: a place for the care of the insane.

Au'ri cle: either of the upper cavities of the heart.

Ba cil'lus: a rodlike bacterium such as the germ of consumption.

Bac te'ri a: tiny one-celled plants often called germs.

Bron'chi (*bron'ki*): the two branches of the windpipe entering the lung.

Bron'chi al: a name given to the small tubes in the lungs.

Cap'il la ry: the smallest blood tube.

Cat'a ract: a growth in the lens of the eye.

Ca tarrh': a common name for a cold in the head.

Cer e bel'lum: the little brain.

Cer'e brum: the large part of the brain.

Chol'e ra in fan'tum: a dangerous disease causing the deaths of about 100,000 children yearly in the United States. It is usually caused by impure milk or dirty milk vessels.

Chyle (*kile*): the digested food in the intestine.

Chyme (*kime*): the partly digested food leaving the stomach.

Cil′i a: tiny hairlike parts of cells lining the nose and air tubes. They catch dust and mucus and move them outward by constantly waving.

Cir cu la′tion: the flow of the blood through the vessels in the body.

Clav′i cle (*klav′i k′l*): the collar bone.

Co′ca ine: a narcotic made from coca leaves.

Coc′cyx (*kok′siks*): the small bone at the end of the spinal column.

Con sti pa′tion: a condition in which the refuse part of the food becomes hard and dry in the lower part of the intestine.

Con ta′gious (*con ta′jus*): catching.

Con vo lu′tions (*con vo lu′shuns*): folds on the surface of the brain.

Cor′ne a: the clear front portion of the outer coat of the eyeball.

Cor′pus cle (*cor′pus s′l*): a blood cell.

Cra′ni um: the bones surrounding the brain.

Di′a phragm (*di′a fram*): the breathing muscle separating the cavity of the chest from that of the abdomen.

Dis in fect′ant: a substance which kills germs.

Dys′en ter y: inflammation of the large intestine with the discharge of some blood.

Dys pep′si a: failure to digest food properly.

Ep i glot′tis: the piece of gristle standing in front of the opening to the larynx.

E soph′a gus (*e sof′a gus*): the tube known as the gullet taking the food from the throat to the stomach.

Ex cre′ta: the natural discharges from the body.

Ex cre′tions: any waste matters cast out of the body.

Fer men ta′tion: the changing of any substance by the growth in it of bacteria, yeasts or molds.

Fis′sure (*fish′ur*): a natural cleft in any organ such as the liver or brain.

For mal′de hyde: a germ-killing gas which is dissolved in water; the solution is then called formalin.

For'ma lin: a good germ killer. A teacupful added to a gallon of water makes a fluid in which any plant or animal may be preserved for years.

Gang'li on: a bunch of nerve cells.

Gar'bage: Waste matter from the kitchen and furnace.

Hy'gi ene: the study of the care of the body.

Im mune': safe from disease.

In cis'ors: the front teeth.

In vol'un ta ry: unable to control.

Lach'ry mal (*lak'ri mal*): the name of the tear gland and its duct into the nose.

Lac'te als: that part of the lymph system leading from the intestines to the thoracic duct.

Lar'ynx (*lar'inks*): the voice box at the top of the trachea.

Lym phat'ics: small tubes known as lymph vessels which return the escaped blood from all parts of the body to the veins in the neck.

Mas sag'ing (*mas sazh'ing*): a kneading and pinching of any part of the body to make the cells work better.

Mi'crobes: bacteria or any other tiny form of life.

Mor'phine: a strong sleep-producing powder derived from opium.

Mu'cous mem'brane: the skinlike lining of all tubes of the body exposed to the air.

Mu'cus: the slippery secretion from the mucous membrane.

Nar cot'ic: a substance which tends to make the organs of the body act more slowly.

Nic'o tine: the chief poison in tobacco.

Ox i da'tion: the union of oxygen with any substance.

Pan'cre as: an organ in the abdomen which makes an important digestive juice.

Pa ral'y sis: loss of power to feel or move in any part.

Par'a site: any plant or animal which eats the living substance of any other plant or animal.

Pa ri'e tal: a bone on the side of the head.

Pas'teur iz ing: heating a substance to about 150 degrees for a half hour or less, sufficient to kill most of the bacteria.

218 PRONUNCIATION AND EXPLANATION OF WORDS

Per i os′te um: the membrane around the bone.

Pha lan′ges (*fa lan′jees*): the bones of the toes and fingers.

Phar′ynx (*far′inks*): the cavity of the throat.

Pro′te id: a substance forming nearly all of muscle after the water is dried out.

Res′pi ra tion: the exchanging of carbon dioxide for oxygen.

Ret′i na: the inner coat of the eye.

Sa′crum: the bone which forms that part of the spinal column between the hips.

Sa li′va: the slippery fluid used in moistening the food in the mouth.

Sew′age: all household waste except the garbage.

Stim′u lant: that which hastens the action of an organ without later slowing it.

Tho rac′ic: belonging to the thorax or chest.

Tib′i a: the larger bone in the lower part of the leg.

Tra′che a (*tra′ke a*): the wind pipe.

Tu ber cu lo′sis: a disease caused by the tubercular germs.

Tym′pa num: the middle ear.

Vac′cine (*vak′sin*): a collection of weak germs or a solution containing a weak poisonous product of germs, put into the body beneath the skin to prevent disease. Smallpox vaccine consists of smallpox germs weakened by growing them in the skin of calves.

Ve′na ca′va: the chief vein in the trunk.

Ven′tri cle: either of the two large lower cavities of the heart.

Ver′te bra: one of the bones of the spinal column.

Vil′li: the tiny fingerlike growths lining the small intestine.

Vit′re ous: the jellylike humor in the back part of the eye.

Vol′un ta ry: able to be controlled by the will.

INDEX

Abdomen, 43.
Adam's apple, 100.
Adenoids, 109, 110, 178.
Air, 95, 98; effect on health, 103–108.
Air sacs, 97.
Albumin, 27.
Alcohol, 18, 30, 34, 46, 55, 57, 66, 76; and blood, 82, 83; and blood vessels, 92; and bones, 142; and brain, 169; and cholera, 198; and clothing, 132; and crime, 69, 172; and digestion, 57, 58; and disease, 196, 197, 198; and eye, 187; and health, 67, 68, 206, 207; and heart, 91; and kidneys, 123, 124; and lungs, 109, 110; and mind, 171; and muscles, 151, 152; and nerves, 170; and pneumonia, 197; and poverty, 68; and skin, 125, 126; and tuberculosis, 110, 198; and warmth, 124, 125.
Alcoholic drink, making of, 62, 63.
Ale, 35.
Alimentary canal, 43, 44, 50–54.
Anatomy, 10.
Antitoxin, 212.
Aorta, 21, 81, 83.
Apoplexy, 164.
Arteries, 81, 84.

Backbone, 21, 136.
Bacteria, 13–16, 32, 80, 122, 123; and disease, 15, 190–196; on fruit, 34; killing of, 38, 40, 44; of milk, 32, 36–38; in water, 61; in wounds, 122, 123.

Bad thoughts, 166.
Baldness, 122.
Bananas, 29.
Barber's itch, 17.
Bathing, 119, 120.
Beans, 33.
Beef, 29, 30, 31, 38, 39.
Beer, 18, 34, 35, 46, 66; and the heart, 92; making of, 64; and the kidneys, 124.
Bile, 55.
Birch beer, 67.
Bladder, 21.
Bleeding, 89, 90.
Blisters, 116.
Blood, 78–91.
Blood corpuscles, 78–80.
Blood plasma, 79, 81.
Blood serum, 79, 81.
Blood vessels, 81–85, 151.
Board of health, 203.
Boils, 15, 195.
Bones, 133–140.
Bone, structure of, 137.
Brain, 155, 157, 161–164; weight of, 165.
Brandy, 46, 65, 66.
Bread, 18, 33.
Breakfast foods, 33.
Breathing, 95–100, 104, 105.
Bronchi, 97.
Bronchial tubes, 97.
Bruises, 122.
Burns and scalds, 123.
Butter, 31, 32.

Cabbage, 29.
Canned meat, 38.

INDEX

Canned fruit, 40.
Capillaries, 82, 85, 97, 151.
Carbon dioxide, 96, 98, 99, 107.
Cartilage, 138.
Cataract, 186.
Catarrh, 108, 109.
Cell, 23, 24.
Cereals, 33.
Cerebellum, 157, 163.
Cerebrum, 161, 163.
Champagne, 65, 66.
Chewing of food, 44, 45, 51.
Chloroform, 172.
Cholera infantum, 37, 196.
Chyle, 53.
Chyme, 51.
Cider, 18, 66, 67.
Cigarettes, 72, 73; and the mind, 168, 169.
Circulation, 88.
Claret, 65, 66.
Cleanliness, 113.
Clothing, 105; and health, 127–131.
Cocaine, 75, 172, 173.
Coffee, 57.
Colds, 128–131; in the head, 108.
Colon, 21.
Constipation, 54.
Consumption, 191–194.
Consumptive, danger from, 210.
Contagious diseases, 188–195.
Corn meal, 28, 29, 33.
Corns, 115, 116.
Cranial nerves, 155.
Cream, 31, 32.
Crystalline lens, 181.
Cucumbers, 29, 57.
Cuts, 122, 123.

Deafness, 178, 179.
Death rate, 11, 13, 188.

Decay, 14.
Dentine, 49.
Diaphragm, 21, 43, 98.
Digestion, in mouth, 44, 45; in stomach, 50, 51; in intestines, 53, 54.
Digestive system, 22, 42–56.
Diphtheria, 11, 15, 16, 37; antitoxin for, 212; deaths from, 188.
Disease, bacteria, 15, 16; cause of, 189–196; germs of, 190; kinds of, 188; prevention of, 200–204.
Dislocation, 141.
Distillation, 65.
Drinking cup and disease, 16, 192, 193.
Drinking water and disease, 60–63, 204.
Dust, 103.
Dying parts, 25.
Dyspepsia, 29, 45.

Ear, 176, 177.
Ears, care of, 178, **179**.
Eating, 56, 57.
Eggs, 30, 31.
Enamel, 49.
Epidermis, 114, **115**.
Epiglottis, 101.
Esophagus, 50.
Ether, 172.
Eye, 180, 181; how weakened, 183, 184; keeping strong, 184.
Eyes, injuries to, 6, 185.
Exercise, 54.
Exercise and health, 150–151, 200.
Exercising the brain, 165; the heart, 89; the lungs, 104; the muscles, 147–149.
Expiration, 98.
Expression, muscles of, 147.

INDEX

Fainting, 89.
Farsightedness, 183.
Fat, 24, 32.
Fats, 28.
Fermentation, 63, 64, 65.
Fever, 11, 15, 37, 60, 61, 195, 196.
Fibrin, 79.
Filtration, 62, 205, 206.
Fish, 29.
Flat chests, 148, 149.
Fleas and disease, 18, 204.
Flies and disease, 193, 201, 204, 205, 209.
Focus, 182.
Food, cooking and care, 36–40; how used in the body, 42–47.
Foods, 27–35.
Formalin, 16, 201, 202, 203.
Fracture, 139, 140.
Fruit, 28, 34, 40.

Gall bladder, 55.
Ganglia, 158.
Garbage, 61.
Gastric glands, 50, 51.
Gastric juice, 51.
Germs, 13–18, 37, 203–206.
Gills, 96.
Ginger ale, 67.
Gland, 42.
Glands, 43, 44, 51.
Grippe, 15.
Gullet, 21, 50.

Habit, 166.
Hair, 121, 122.
Headache, 34, 45.
Headache powders, 76.
Health officer, 203
Hearing, 176–178.
Heart, 21, 81, 83, 84, 88.
Heat, regulation of, 117, 118.

Hipjoint disease, 194.
Hygiene, 10, 11.

Ice water, 60.
Indigestion, 29, 45, 57.
Inflammation, 195.
Insects and disease, 18, 193, 195, 201, 204, 205, 209, 214.
Inspiration, 98.
Intestines, 21, 52–54.
Itch, 18, 19.

Joints, 140.

Kidney, 21, 113, 123.

Lacteals, 53, 54, 55.
Lard, 28.
Larynx, 96, 100, 101.
Laudanum, 75, 76.
Length of life, 12.
Leprosy, 15.
Lice, 18, 19.
Ligaments, 140, 141.
Lister, 123.
Liver, 21, 52, 53, 54, 55, 56.
Lockjaw, 15, 195.
Lymph nodes, 87.
Lymph vessels, 86, 87.
Lungs, 21, 96, 97; care of, 103–105.

Malaria, 15, 196.
Malt liquors, 64.
Meats, 30, 31, 34, 38–39.
Medulla oblongata, 163.
Meningitis, 194.
Microbes, 13–18.
Milk, 12, 28, 31, 33, 36–38.
Milk teeth, 47, 48, 50.
Mind, 165–167.
Mineral matter, 27, 34.
Mold, 16, 17.

Morphine, 74, 75.
Mosquitoes and disease, 195, 196, 203, 214.
Mucous membrane, 44, 51.
Mucus, 44.
Muscle fiber, 143.
Muscles, 143–149.
Muscles, kinds of, 146.

Nails, care of, 120, 121.
Narcotic, 69.
Narcotics, 71–77.
Narcotics and sense organs, 186.
Nearsightedness, 183.
Nerve cell, 24, 155, 158.
Nerves, 153–158.
Nerves, endings of, 174, 175.
Nervous system, 153–173.
Nicotine, 72.
Nitrogen, 95.
Nursing bottle, 37.

Oatmeal, 33.
Oil, 28.
Opium, 74.
Organs of the body, 21, 22, 43.
Oxidation, 25, 96.
Oxygen, 25, 95, 98, 99.
Oysters, 29.

Pancreas, 21, 52, 53, 54, 55.
Paralysis, 163.
Parasites, 18–20, 188.
Paregoric, 75, 76.
Pasteurizing, 38, 204.
Patent medicines, 66, 76, 77.
Periosteum, 138.
Physiology, 10.
Plague, 204.
Pneumonia, 15, 191; deaths from, 188.
Potatoes, 29.

Proteid, 27, 28, 31.
Pulse, 88.

Reflex action, 160.
Respiration, 99.
Ribs, 133, 135.
Ringworm, 17.
Round shoulders, 148, 149.

Saliva, 44, 191.
Salivary glands, 44.
Scarf skin, 115.
Scarlet fever, 37.
Scrofula, 194.
Scurvy, 11.
Secretion, 43.
Senses, 174–181.
Sewage, 61.
Shoes and health, 131.
Sick, caring for, 202.
Sickness, prevention of, 213.
Sick room, 203.
Sight, 180, 182.
Sirloin, 29, 30.
Skin, 114, 121, 175.
Skull, 134, 136.
Sleep, 167.
Sleeping sickness, 15, 18.
Smallpox, 10, 211, 212.
Smell, 175.
Smoking tobacco, 72, 73.
Smoking, effect on eyes, 186.
Snuff, 74.
Soda water, 67.
Soft drinks, 67.
Soothing syrup, 75, 76.
Sore throat, 15, 16.
Soups, 33.
Spinal column, 136.
Spinal cord, 154, 158–160.
Spinal nerves, 157.
Spleen, 21, 52.

INDEX

Spore, 16, 17.
Sprain, 141.
Starch, 28.
Stimulant, 69.
Stomach, 50, 51.
Strain, 141.
Sugars, 28.
Sweat, 127, 128.
Sweat glands, 114, 118.
Sympathetic nerves, 157, 158, 159.
Systems, 22.

Tallow, 28.
Tanning and freckles, 116, 117.
Taste, 176.
Tea, 57.
Teeth, 47–50.
Tendons, 144, 145.
Thoracic duct, 54, 86.
Tissues, 22, 23.
Tobacco, 45, 71–74; and blood, 93; and bones, 142; and lungs, 110, 111; and muscles, 151; and nerves, 167.
Tonsilitis, 37.
Tonsils, 101, 109, 110, 189.
Toothbrush, 49.
Trachea, 96, 97.
Tuberculosis, 15, 16, 38, 68; and alcohol, 110, 198; cause of, 191–194; in cows, 193; cure of,

Tuberculosis.—*Continued*
209, 210; deaths from, 188, 208; germs of, 15; prevention of, 207–209.
Typhoid fever, 15, 37, 60, 61; germs of, 194; cause of, 37, 194, 195; prevention of, 204.

Vaccination, 211, 212.
Vegetables, 30, 33, 39.
Veins, 81, 82, 84.
Vena cava, 54.
Ventilation, 105–108.
Vertebræ, 134, 136.
Villi, 52–55.
Vocal cords, 100, 101.
Voice, 101, 102.

Warts, 116.
Water, bacteria in, 13, 14; in the body, 27; drinking of, 57; in food, 31, 33; and health, 60–62.
Wheat, 28, 29.
Whisky, 46, 65, 66, 82.
White swelling, 194.
Wine, 18, 57, 64, 65.
Windpipe, 21, 96, 97.
Wounds, care of, 90, 91.

Yeast, 17, 18, 63.
Yellow fever, 18, 196, 214.